Talk With Me

Experiences with Autism in the LDS Community

Compiled by:
Kathy Weatherford
and
Natalie Wright

authorHOUSE™

1663 LIBERTY DRIVE, SUITE 200
BLOOMINGTON, INDIANA 47403
(800) 839-8640
WWW.AUTHORHOUSE.COM

First published by AuthorHouse 07/11/05

ISBN: 1-4208-7143-9 (e)
ISBN: 1-4208-5769-X (sc)

Printed in the United States of America
Bloomington, Indiana

This book is printed on acid-free paper.

Dedication

For all of the people we love, for all of the family and friends who were supportive—most especially our fabulous editor, Amy Redmon (many thankful hugs, Mom!), and for all of our precious children, we dedicate this, our effort to help other families deal with autism by giving them the best thing we can, our experiences. May all who read this be touched by the Holy Spirit and have a new resolve and tools to be accepting, helpful, and loving to the ones you know who have autism and the ones you know who are living with autism in their homes.

Contents

Introduction

by Meg Stout

You may be wondering why there is a book about autism in the Mormon (or Latter-day Saint) community. I doubt any credible scientist would hypothesize that the rate of autism is affected by family belief system. So we may assume that, among Mormons just as in the general population, autism or some other developmental delay on the autism spectrum affects 1 person out of 160,[1] with the rate of incidence on the rise.[2]

But it is not the rate of incidence that warrants a book on autism among Mormons. Rather, the Mormon experience does make any significant life experience different. Most of the experiences in this book could happen to anyone dealing with an autistic child. But here and there you will see the authors describe either anguish or peace because of circumstances and beliefs that are not common to other cultures. In this chapter, I'd like to give you a brief introduction to some of those circumstances (Mormon church organization and culture) and beliefs (Mormon theology).

How the organization and culture of the Church of Jesus Christ of Latter-day Saints (i.e., the Mormon church) affects the experience of having an autistic family member

There are three major ways in which Mormon organization and culture differ from other faith traditions: how congregations are formed, how leaders are selected and trained, and how members of the congregation interact. This doesn't account for every unique Mormon trait. For example, I'm not sure what these three factors have to do with the pre-eminence of green Jell-O in Mormon desserts. But I think the reader will find these factors account for much of the confusion a non-Mormon might experience reading this book.

---

[1] "Pervasive Developmental Disorders in Preschool Children", Suniti Chakrabarti, MD, MRCP; Eric Fombonne, MD, FRCPsych, Journal of the American Medical Association, vol. 285, p. 3093, June 27, 2001.

[2] "M.I.N.D. Institute Study Confirms Autism Increase", Oct. 17, 2002, News from UC Davis Health System [online] available at http://news.ucdmc.ucdavis.edu/mindepi_study.html,11 Nov 2002. California has seen a 273% increase in incidence of autism from 1987 to 1998, which cannot be wholly accounted for by better diagnoses and an increase in the general population.

Formation of Mormon congregations. Unlike most other religious congregations, Mormons are organized centrally, and you attend a congregation (ward or branch) based on your geographical location. This means a Mormon can move almost anywhere in the world and know which congregation they are to attend, whether in Kazakhstan, India, or the United States. I have known of families to make housing decisions based on which congregation they would belong to at that address. In other religions, the influence of the pastor or priest has a lot to do with whether the congregation withers or flourishes, and congregations can grow to include thousands or even tens of thousands of worshippers. A Mormon congregation cannot grow very large without being 'reorganized', with congregational boundaries realigned until all the congregations in that area are again sized according to world-wide church guidelines.

What does any of this have to do with autism? Well, it means that a Mormon who wishes to change congregations can't legitimately start attending a different congregation, other than by doing something as drastic as moving. And the church guidelines maintain congregations at approximately 200-300 families, or 500-800 individuals. Based on this size, it is likely that any given Mormon congregation will include an autistic individual, but at most only a few autistic individuals. This can result in an opportunity for an entire congregation to know the autistic individuals in their midst and care for their particular needs. But it also means that most everyone in that congregation is dealing with those autistic individuals from a relatively uninformed standpoint, putting a burden for education on the family of the autistic individual.

Lay Leadership. A unique aspect of Mormonism is the absence of a paid clergy. I could write volumes about the general pros (and cons) of lay leadership versus paid clergy. The great thing is that the ability to fill any position in the congregation is only limited by the membership of the congregation. The bad thing is that the ability to fill any position in the congregation is limited to the membership of the congregation!

With respect to autism, this ability to call on the entire talent pool of a congregation can be an excellent thing. In my own case, this has resulted in my daughter's being helped at church by people whose work-a-day job is special education. However, some have found that leaders in their congregations are uninformed or overloaded by families and jobs in addition to their church responsibilities.

Another aspect of the lay ministry in the Mormon Church is the great flexibility this can provide. There are no 'career paths' in the church, so the right person can be called upon to help where they are needed, when they are needed, without regard for any negative impact this might have of their future "church career." This flexibility can be great for parents of autistic children when it is used to help those children. Periodic training, mentoring by senior leaders and 1-800 numbers staffed by professionals help compensate for lack of formal pastoral education. But it can be bewildering when leaders in the congregation choose not to reach out to our sometimes-difficult children.

All families of children with disabilities deal with these pros and cons of lay leadership. But I suspect that it may be a bit more difficult for those dealing with autism. Autistic individuals rarely look different from other children. The sympathy and understanding that would be accorded to a child with an obvious challenge, such as Down's Syndrome, is not immediately forthcoming for these perfect looking children who refuse to talk and behave and potty train and "be reverent." And there is no medication that necessarily mitigates autistic behavior, like there is for conditions such as Attention Deficit Hyperactivity Disorder (ADHD).

A Peculiar People. Mormons build and maintain tight-knit communities. This is in part due to history. Early Mormons were subjected to "untolled hardship and trauma" east of the Mississippi during the 1830's and 1840's.[3] After leaving Illinois, the Mormons fled to the mountainous west—a harsh and arid place where community cooperation was critical to survival. Even though far fewer than 50% of modern Mormons are descended from 19th-century Mormons, the culture and practices of the modern church continue to emphasize community and interpersonal support.

One aspect of a tight-knit community is the pressure to norm. Unfortunately, autistic people just don't fit the norm. In fact, part of the autism complex is the lack of the usual need to meet social norms. For families of an autistic individual, the inability to be 'normal' can be painful, either due to internal perceptions or external criticism.

On the positive side, each family has several sets of people assigned to watch out for them. Each family is assigned a pair of men (home teachers) who are supposed to visit each month, and each adult woman is assigned

---

[3] See resolution HR0627 passed by the 93rd Illinois General Assembly in March 2004 apologizing for hardship and trauma the community of Latter-day Saints (Mormons) suffered because of distrust, violence, and inhospitable actions of a dark time in the past of the State of Illinois, available online [25 Jan 2005] at http://www.ilga.gov/legislation/default.asp?ga=93.

a pair of women to contact them each month. Even children can expect their Sunday School teacher or Young Men/Young Women advisors to reach out to them specifically.

Beyond receiving services from the community, being able to offer service to others can be a great comfort, even for the overburdened families of autistic individuals. In fact, being denied the opportunity to participate in the community can in itself cause great pain, even if intended to provide relief to overburdened parents of autistic children.

How the theology of the Mormon Church affects the experience of having an autistic family member

In my professional life, one of my major tasks is to "manage expectations." Finding oneself immersed in mud takes on a very different meaning if it is in the context of a high-priced spa rather than at the side of a road in a cold rainstorm. Mormon theology has a huge impact on what believers expect it means to have a loved one with autism. First, Mormons believe we existed before conception or any physical or mental handicaps, that we are beloved spirit children of God. Next, Mormonism puts much significance on the choices, service and family opportunities we have in this life. Finally, Mormons have distinct expectations of the life after death – much more concrete than a mere hope for an afterlife.

Children of God. Mormonism is a theology of great hope. One of the first songs Mormon children learn is "I am a Child of God." Mormons believe that each individual is an eternal being or intelligence. God gives these "intelligences" spiritual life, making us all, in fact, spirit children of God, or Heavenly Father. God then offers his spirit children the opportunity to be born into physical life, or the life we have on this earth. Thus, we are not creations of some distant, unknowable being, but beloved children of a caring (if omniscient and omnipotent) God.

Mormons understand this life as a time to gain a physical body and to prove who we really are when we are not under constant divine instruction and direction. In keeping with God's personal involvement with each and every one of us, Mormons believe that all individuals born on this earth will be resurrected, even those who prove by their unrepentant evil acts that they do not wish to have anything to do with God. In the resurrection we will all be raised again in incorruptible, perfect bodies. No blindness, no deafness, no lameness. No autism.

Baptism. Mormons believe that part of the purpose of this life is to prove by our choices that we do love God and God's work. A tangible and necessary symbol of our love for God is the decision to join God's church via baptism. Because the decision to be baptized must be a conscious choice, Mormons are not baptized until they are capable of making this choice. This "age of accountability" is eight years of age for people who are neurologically typical. For those who die before they are mentally capable of making this choice, Christ's atonement pays for their transgressions. And proxy baptism can be performed on behalf of those who died without proper baptism, which baptism would be either accepted or rejected by the deceased prior to judgment day.

In the case of some autistic individuals, they are able to choose, but unable to communicate their choice. In this special and unique instance, the person is not to be baptized. This can be hard for a family who "just knows" that the child wants to be baptized. It can also be hard for convert families who feel that an un-baptized child will be damned. Even when an autistic individual can communicate, it can be difficult to figure out when they are actually accountable.

Priesthood and Missionary Service. Since a significant majority of autistic individuals are male, it is worth mentioning the effect autism can have on priesthood and priesthood service. All worthy, baptized men may receive the priesthood starting at age 12. When an autistic man is unable to receive the priesthood with his age-peers (because he has not yet been baptized), it is a renewed symbol that things are not right, and can be a source of distress. Some church activities for the young men involve service which only priesthood holders may perform, such as collection of donations for the needy (fast offerings) and the weekly preparation and distribution of the sacrament. Autistic boys who cannot receive the priesthood can become further isolated from their peers, and their families can become further isolated from the rest of the congregation.

Perhaps the most significant rite of passage for young Mormon men is missionary service—two years spent teaching people about the gospel of Jesus Christ at their own or their family's expense. For the past several decades, missionary service has been expected of all young men. [Missionary service from women is appreciated but not expected.] Missionaries no longer go "without purse or scrip," depending entirely on those they teach for their sustenance and shelter. However, missionary service is still very demanding; physically, spiritually, socially and financially. Having been a missionary, I can understand how difficult or impossible it would be to be a successful missionary in the face of autism. Understanding, spiritual depth and physical strength are not sufficient - one must be able to successfully relate to and work with a previously unknown 19-20 year old, 24 hours a day, 7 days a week. When a young Mormon man fails to serve a mission or returns home early, uninformed associates can jump to unflattering conclusions. This can be an opportunity to remind people that sexual sin is not the only bar to missionary service. Since the church does not pay missionaries, most autistic individuals are relieved of a financial commitment that other young Mormon men and their families are making. But it causes many Mormon families sorrow when it becomes clear that a child will be unable to fulfill a mission.

Marriage. In 1845, the Mormon poetess Eliza R. Snow penned "In the heavens, are parents single? No, the thought makes reason stare. Truth is reason, truth eternal tells me I've a mother there." Since the early days of Mormonism, marriage has been very important. In Mormon scripture, God states, "This is My Work and My Glory - to bring to pass the immortality and eternal life of man." We've discussed how Mormons believe that God grants all peoples resurrection and life throughout eternity, otherwise known as immortality. "Eternal life" is understood to be the highest glory and honor we can achieve, and consists of being with God and assisting Him in His work. Marriage, particularly temple marriage for eternity, is therefore very important in Mormonism, for only those who have a partner in eternity are understood to be able to perform the function of giving spiritual birth in the eternities.

The doctrinally based emphasis on marriage can have various effects on families dealing with autism. Dealing with an autistic child can cause great strain, and I believe studies in the general population show a correlation between having an autistic child and an increased probability of divorce. These strains also occur in LDS families, and Mormon families are not immune to divorce. However, the doctrine of eternal marriage gives a reason for staying together when the stress is great.

The communication difficulties of those with autism result in much lower chance of such individuals marrying, or of the marriage succeeding [Nash, J. Madeline, "The Secrets of Autism," May 6, 2002, *Time* [online] available at http://www.time.com/time/covers/1101020506]. In addition, the strong genetic component of autism means children of autistic individuals are far more likely to experience pervasive developmental delays than the 1/160 rate seen in the general population. Mormon theology provides hope that eternal marriage can occur, even for those who never married in life. But it is hard to suspect or know that mortal marriage is impossible for a loved one who is autistic. Again there can be pain from internal expectations or external criticism.

Eternal Life. Baptism, missionary service and marriage may not be reasonable expectations for many autistic individuals in this life. But Mormons expect that all will be resurrected and restored to bodies that are free from defects such as autism. No one will be denied eternal life because of circumstances beyond their control. Though there can be many disappointments in this life when our autistic family members are unable to progress with their age-peers, Mormons believe that at some future date these individuals will be freed from the neural abnormalities that isolate them from us in this life. To paraphrase St. Paul, at that day our children shall be delivered from the bondage of autism and be welcomed into the glorious liberty of the children of God. [c.f. Rom 8:21]

Summary

I've attempted to cover the major ways being Mormon affects the experience of dealing with autism, both for good and ill. I hope this information will help you better understand the experiences you will read about in this book. Most of all, I hope you will be better able to learn from and appreciate the joys, sorrows, and challenges you will see through the eyes of these authors.

Chapter One

Matthew, age 2
By Natalie Wright

Natalie Wright was born and raised in Sandy, Utah. She moved to Maine in 1999 and currently resides in Kennebunk with her husband and two children. Natalie graduated from Ricks College with an associates degree in Fine Arts and Photography. In 2002 she founded SquarePics, a company dedicated to helping children with speech delays and disorders to communicate. Her products are currently used all over the nation. In 2003 Natalie created and developed a website with resources for LDS parents and educators working with special needs children (www.squarepics.com/lds). Natalie enjoys in her free time scrapbooking, photography, reading, and spending time with her family. Her son Matthew was diagnosed with autistic spectrum disorder.

My husband Dallan and I consider ourselves immensely blessed with our two children and a beautiful, simple home in Kennebunk, Maine. We live in a small town with quiet neighbors. The beaches are only two miles east; shops and delicious seafood are two miles to the west. The winters are dry and cold, the summers warm and humid; but we always find a chance to escape to the ocean. We feel at home in New England. We feel it is a wonderful place to rear our children.

As I think back to when both of our children were born, I recall how perfect they both seemed. We were so excited about Taylor, our first; she was so beautiful. Although her head was squashed like a cone, she looked perfect to me—and after a few days perfect to the rest of the world as well. She was born on a cold day in November, and Matthew came just eighteen months later, in May. Another beautiful, perfect baby! He looked just like a miniature version of his father (minus the facial hair). His head was covered in long, thick, black hair—a big surprise after his blond, bald sister! He even had his father's adorable, "squashed" chin.

Just as Taylor did, Matthew seemed to grow and develop perfectly. We were always a little concerned with his noticeable reflux (he seemed to spit up and vomit all the time); but we read that reflux was all completely normal for a young, healthy baby. He seemed to grow out of it around his first birthday. When he was one and a half, his problem with reflux returned.

He suddenly began vomiting constantly, throwing up everything from milk and juice to bland foods (like crackers). First, the vomiting was only once every few days, then two or three times a day, and back and forth again. It seemed to peak at nineteen months (around Christmas time) when he began throwing up several times a day. We blamed it on everything: being on vacation, or maybe jet lag, or being off his normal routine. But when we came home, his vomiting continued to worsen. We sought out advice, sharing our frustration with friends, only to hear that their child went through the same thing, or that it was normal, or that he would eventually grow out of it. I insisted on visiting the pediatrician, feeling on the verge of a breakdown. If, in fact, all this vomiting was normal, then I would take it in stride; but it seemed to me to be worth checking out! He agreed, discussed a few ideas, and sent us home with an over-the-counter Pepcid AC medication.

Taylor was now starting to sense my tension and worry. On one occasion we had arrived late to church and had to sit in the only available pew near the front of the chapel. Matthew was happily lining up his toy cars on the bench, as he always did, and he let out a loud, coughing sneeze. Taylor turned to me and, with her loud three-year-old voice, asked, "Is Maffew going to frow up, Mommy?"

Dallan and I quickly shushed her and sank in our seats. Several members of the congregation glanced at us, wondering why we would bring a child to church with the flu.

Matthew and Taylor always attended the nursery after sacrament meeting on Sundays. Although he was attached to us and disliked going by himself, Matthew enjoyed the lessons and toys, and seeing the other children. The nursery teacher approached us one Sunday to inform us that he had been upset and had cried—and that he had vomited all over the floor. She was patient and didn't seem annoyed, but we were embarrassed just the same. We quickly cleaned up the mess. He began vomiting all the time during the nursery and other church meetings. When we explained he did it randomly and was not sick, most people smiled and were supportive—giving us their advice.

Two weeks later I was back at the pediatrician's office with Matthew. He seemed to be eating twice as much food as he was vomiting; so he was probably getting enough nourishment; but he had still visibly lost some weight. His doctor put Matthew on a stronger medication and ordered an upper GI test at the local hospital. We prayed the test would find what was causing all the discomfort and vomiting. We spent hours wondering what might be causing all this turmoil in his little tummy.

The test was dreadful! Dallan and I both accompanied Matthew to the hospital. We had to arrive early in the morning, and we were all three exhausted from lack of sleep. At twenty months old, he was still waking up for a bottle in the night. Since he was not allowed to eat for eight hours before the test, he was miserable and starving. We ended up fighting to deal with his screaming and crying, as we waited and waited. Besides his being hungry, he seemed so nervous about being in this strange, new place.

The testing finally began with some simple chest x-rays. Then we were sent back to the waiting room again. When it was finally his turn again, I was sweating and shaking from nerves and anger. Dallan was not allowed to accompany me, and we both gave each other a look of "why did we go to all the work to find a sitter?"

I followed a petite nurse into a large, dark room that would have scared even me. A long, thin table was in the middle of the room; and a gigantic, black box hung directly over it. I looked around to find two more nurses and the doctor watching me. They were covered in what looked like pastel, bullet-proof vests that covered their torsos up to their necks.

Matthew clung to my hair and shirt as I stripped off his clothing. They could have at least warmed the room for my son; it was freezing. They finally produced a bottle full of white, chalky barium; and he almost leapt out of my arms to get it. The bottle was the only possible comfort he found in the room, and he gladly gulped down the substance.

It made me sick watching him drink it. It must have tasted awful, but he gladly swallowed it down. He was allowed to drink about a third of the bottle and then he was placed on top of the metal table, which was cold to the touch. I was glad he had worked up a sweat fighting and crying. The doctor pulled the large box down almost on top of him. Matthew looked so small and helpless underneath it. It was about his length, and three times his width. His eyes peered helplessly up at me as I stood above his head, out of the way.

The doctor began explaining what he was going to do, and I wondered why he hadn't done that before my son was held down on a cold table against his will. Before the doctor began photographing, I quickly questioned whether I should wear a pastel, bullet- proof vest myself. The nurses blushed and rushed to give me one twice the size of theirs, with a piece that wrapped around my neck like a scarf. Matthew screamed and arched his back as I turned away from him to put it on. He helplessly looked at me, as if he thought I was going to leave him—as if I wanted to torture him even more.

Throughout the whole process he never did calm down. The doctor simply yelled over the top of him, telling me what a great wrestler Matthew would be one day. The crew took what seemed like a hundred x-rays, and I was finally allowed to pick up my son. A few minutes later the doctor returned to let me know he was sorry but he needed to take a few more shots on an area he questioned. This time Matthew and I both cried together, as my son was once again held down against both his will and mine.

Three days later our pediatrician's nurse Carol gave us a call with results. I had always loved and appreciated our pediatrician, but there was something extra about Carol's voice that always brought comfort to me whenever we were dealing with sick children.

On the phone she sighed, sounding as frustrated as I had been over the last few weeks. The news seemed good; nothing was found on the test. But the only problem was that the test showed he had absolutely no sign of reflux. The vomiting was caused by something else entirely!

It took Matthew several days to overcome the anxiety of the visit to the hospital. He seemed to have a scowl on his face for a week; but he eventually forgave me and we went on as normal, playing, laughing, and cleaning vomit off the floors.

Our pediatrician informed us that this ordeal was out of his hands, and he sent us to a pediatric gastroenterologist. By the time we went to this specialist, almost a month had passed; and Matthew had improved dramatically on his current, prescribed medication. It seemed not only to control all the acid in his stomach, but also to strengthen his esophagus and intestines as well. He was still vomiting occasionally, but we rejoiced in the improvement and were willing to live with the occasional clean up, if we had to. We still did not understand what was going on in his little body; so with both kids I drove the thirty miles north to the specialist to see if we might find some answers.

The doctor's office was very small, and we were the only patients in sight—besides a small girl who sat across from us. I hoped Taylor wouldn't notice her and say anything embarrassing. She was obviously handicapped and had some serious health problems. Although it was hard to tell her age by looking at her, she seemed to be about five. Her stomach was large and bloated, compared to her tiny body. Her face was flat and distorted, and she wore thick glasses on her wide nose. She seemed quiet and unfocused as she sat on her mother's lap. I felt selfish for bringing in my son who looked perfectly healthy to the human eye.

The doctor's visit was short. We reviewed Matthew's case and discussed his current heath and medication. Even though we were still unsure about the cause of the vomiting, the doctor thought he possibly just had a very bad gag reflex and had trouble controlling the acid in his stomach. We planned to have Matt return in a few months, and we both had high hopes for his health and recovery. Although he threw up all over the car on the way home, I tried to tell myself that I would too after being poked and prodded by the doctor.

The medicine continued to work wonders. Matthew was not only vomiting less, but seemed over all to feel better. He no longer winced in stomach pain and looked uncomfortable. He was able to start sleeping on his own again. Even if he still did wake for a bottle in the night, we figured it was just out of habit. We gave in to him out of gratitude for having clean beds.

We continued on with our happy lives for the next month, reporting to everyone we knew that Matthew was doing well again. The nursery at church gladly took him in, accepting that he still might vomit once in a while. We started attending more church activities and spending more time with friends. I signed up the kids for several toddler classes through our town's Parks and Recreational Department. We also found a few play groups we could attend in town. I thought the time with other kids and moms would be good for all of us. It was finally spring! Although the air was still cool, we were getting out of the house more and seemed to be enjoying ourselves.

A few weeks after Matthew's visit to the specialist, my mother came to visit. She too had noticed the improvement in Matthew's vomiting, and together we rejoiced in his better health. Although Matthew was now throwing up less, my mother expressed some concern about his development and speech being delayed. He had never spoken before (except a few times where I think he might have said "Dad" and "dog"), and we had always thought he was just a little behind. After all that vomiting who would be talking fluently? I assumed his esophagus was damaged and needed some time to heal. He was making some simple sounds such as da, do, and ish but had never put together a complete word that seemed to mean anything. He was now twenty-two months, so I focused even harder on helping him speak.

While my mother was visiting, there was one thing about Matthew I couldn't help but notice. He had a very difficult time with her presence and would get upset every time she drew near him. He did not want to be touched by her and would not look at her. He has always been a little shy, but he knew my mother well and had let her hold him in the past. He cried and repeatedly hit his head on the floor when she came near. Yet when Dallan and I spent a night out in Boston, he seemed to be fine with her. He never let her hold him, but never cried for us; he just kept to himself. I was shocked by this new behavior. I had never seen a child hit his head out of anger or frustration. I started noticing other changes in Matthew as well. He no longer seemed to connect with Taylor. He acted as if she wasn't in the room, and he would not play with her. He started doing the same head-banging when she would come near.

I began to wonder if Matthew's history of vomiting was at all related to this new behavior, but I dismissed that idea due to his amazing recovery and decrease in vomiting. I began searching the Internet for information about relationships between vomiting and delays in learning. I found nothing; but I did come across a few things that related to his behavior. What I found was called PDD (Pervasive Developmental Disorder). It was the umbrella over many developmental disorders such as Rhett's Syndrome, Asperger's Syndrome, fragile-X syndrome, and autism. I had heard of these before but knew nothing about them. I dismissed them all immediately; Matthew wasn't like any of these. He was just fine and would grow out of this phase. My visiting mother soon returned home, and I thought that our being back to routine would help Matthew.

He slowly continued to worsen. His simple toddler behaviors dwindled as he withdrew into himself more and more. He loved being outdoors; but instead of playing in our home-built playhouse or kicking around a ball, he would just run in circles or back and forth all over the yard. He would occasionally look back to see if I was following him but then eventually ignored me and ran as fast as he could, back and forth between our yard and the neighbors' yards. He suddenly had no sense of danger, and I found I had to follow his every step to keep him away from the nearby road and neighbors' dogs.

His love for running became an obsession, as he would bolt for freedom every time we opened the front door. He would look up at the sky as he ran forward, kicking his knees up as he ran. He would never look back and would continue as fast as he could go. He was a chore at the beach, running almost a mile down the coast before we finally convinced him to head in the other direction. Sometimes we ended up carrying him screaming back to the car. He was so difficult to watch compared to Taylor, who loved to just sit and play peacefully. She was often neglected by me, since I was so preoccupied with chasing her brother around the yard.

Matthew also had always loved music, but he no longer showed interest in banging on a drum or shaking a maraca. He seemed suddenly to despise my singing, which had soothed him as a baby. He would throw himself from my arms and bang his head every time I began a familiar tune. He seemed to like some noise, and he would spin in circles in the kitchen every time I turned on the dishwasher, dryer, or vacuum.

Matthew always seemed to find some peace with his toy cars. He loved them more than anything. When his grandfather had visited in the past Matthew would sit on his lap for hours looking through books about cars from the library. He still seemed to be obsessed with toy cars, but he suddenly seemed to play with them differently. Instead of driving them around, he would line them all up, each facing the right direction in a perfect parking lot formation. He did this for hours and hours. He would move them from one side of the room to another, each time placing them in a straight line. I would try to throw him off by turning one to face backwards, and he would immediately correct me or bang his head on the floor in disapproval. When I took him shopping, he no longer cared about picking out a new car at the store. He just stared ahead at the lights and movement around us.

He began displaying all of his strange new habits away from home, banging his head at play groups and withdrawing from the other kids in the group. At church he was impossible, running the circular halls during the long meeting hours. We were afraid to send him to the nursery since he might bang his head and hurt himself. They didn't seem to understand this new behavior anyway.

I searched for more about developmental disorders and finally suggested to my husband the possibility of Matthew's having a disorder. I even mentioned the word autism. He shrugged at my suggestion; but at the end of the day, after searching autism out on the Internet, he came home from work convinced Matthew had the disorder. He had printed out a list of symptoms and placed small checks next to the ones that Matt was displaying. Almost every item had been checked.

I openly discussed the symptoms with him, but I was still very skeptical afterwards because Matthew lacked what I thought was one of the major symptoms: no eye contact. Even though he would not look at others, he still made eye contact with me. He would not look at me for long, but he would still occasionally glance when I held up a toy or spoke to him. For heaven sakes, he even smiled at me! If he were autistic, surely he would not be doing this.

A friend soon referred me to a group who was supplying speech therapy for her immature daughter. I figured Matthew would grow out of his new behaviors, but definitely would benefit from a speech therapist, since he still wasn't talking. The speech therapists then referred me to Child Developmental Services, a state-funded service for helping children with delays. We set up an assessment for Matthew. As we waited weeks for the assessment, Matthew withdrew more and more. I attended fewer play groups and classes due to the looks I was receiving every time he would bang his head or spin in circles. I was embarrassed, but not by his behavior—just by the fact I didn't know why he was doing it. I could not explain it.

I had finally had enough when at one class a toddler about half Matt's size, and at least six months younger, came and spontaneously sat directly on my lap alongside Matthew. He had no fear of joining us and looked directly into my eyes. He was curious about the book I was trying to read to my squirming toddler, who just wanted to sit by himself and flip the pages back and forth. I was happily surprised, and since the boy's mother was busy across the room, encouraged him to join us. He seemed so alert and aware of me (compared to Matthew who was still fighting his way off my lap). I freed my arm and let Matthew run, focusing on the toddler still in my lap. I'll see how normal Matthew is. I'll test this kid. I smiled at him and pointed to the book in my lap.

"Do you know what this is?" I said, pointing to the picture on the front cover. "Ish," he replied. This was a sound Matthew had made in the past; but to this child, the word obviously had a meaning, since he pointed to the brightly colored fish on the page. I thought I would try a harder question: "What color is the fish?"

"Wed."

Okay, he knows one color. "What color is the seaweed?" I hoped he didn't even know what seaweed was.

"Seaweed is gween".

Damn. He knew that one, too. By now Matthew was running at full speed around the room in circles. I looked for a tougher book. We lived on the coast; of course this kid knows a little oceanography. I found one to meet his match, an older child's book full of trucks and cars. "Do you know these colors too?" I asked sarcastically.

"Dat's bwoo, lellow, and pewple."

He proudly stood up and walked away to find another child to play with. To make myself feel better, I told myself his mother would need a speech therapist for him one day too.

As we waited for Matthew's assessment, we continued to worry about other things—such as his lost coordination to drink from a regular cup. He would oddly extend his tongue all the way when trying to get a drink from my glass. He had forgotten how to close his lips around the glass, so the liquid would rush down his shirt as I tried to help him get a drink. He had never liked using silverware but definitely knew how. Now he would not touch silverware and insisted on only eating finger foods. His diet changed dramatically. Although it was easy just to feed him chicken nuggets, French fries, and dry cereal, I wondered why he would no longer eat yogurt, mashed potatoes, and other soft foods he had once loved.

He also seemed to develop a strange obsession with hair and string. We often found him playing with loose hair and eating pieces of string off the floor. I gave up sewing for a while when I found him perched at the top of my desk in front of my sewing machine, feeding himself the thread right off the bobbin. He had a mouthful by the time I pulled him down. Then he screamed and banged his head on the floor. I had to vacuum constantly (which he enjoyed, since he spun in circles whenever I turned the vacuum on).

Over the next few days I became obsessed, using all of my free time studying developmental disorders. The more I read, the more I was convinced that Matthew was autistic. I even discovered that children's not making eye contact was a myth about autism. Some children indeed could look at you, smile, laugh, and be happy. The drive to learn more kept me up late at night and woke me early in the morning. I would wake at five or six with Matthew; but after he sipped his bottle back to "dream world," I would lie in bed agitated, my mind racing, unable to go back to sleep.

9

The phone was ringing off the hook. More and more family members who had heard of Matt's troubles, called. They all were polite and wished us well, but I found it difficult to explain the situation over and over again, when I myself didn't understand it. A friend called, and since I had been avoiding the phone all day, I finally decided to answer. After some small talk I filled her in on Matt's recent behaviors. She had not seen Matthew for several weeks, and she was very surprised by my concerns. I told her of some of Matt's recent new habits and behaviors. She paused, then replied that he had always seemed fine to her; and although she thought his speech a little slow, overall he seemed just fine. When I finally suggested the word autism, she exploded in laughter on the phone and firmly told me that Matthew did NOT have autism.

She had studied special education in college and proceeded to tell me she had worked with many autistic children, who were nothing like Matthew. I tried to explain (although I deeply wanted to believe her) that Matthew had regressed since she last saw him and was showing many of the signs that autistic children have. She obviously did not believe me. After some lame excuse, I was finally able to get off the phone.

Were other people laughing at my assumptions? I felt furious and betrayed. I thought a mother's instinct was always right, and I had some good reasons for being concerned. I never expected anyone not to believe me. Was I just paranoid? I began wishing no one knew what we thought and that I had never discovered autism. I wanted to crawl under the coffee table where Matthew was now lying, staring off into space.

I bent over and pulled him out, knowing he must be tired. It was almost four in the afternoon, and his naps were getting later and later. I took him into the kitchen and held him in my arms. I began to sing a soft lullaby until he started squirming and fighting me. I ceased singing, and he settled down again. After he swayed back and forth for awhile, I realized he was not going to give in, and I gave up giving him a bottle and put him down on the couch. Looking off into the distance, Matthew slowly closed his eyes and dreamt of the warm milk trickling down his throat.

I climbed the stairs to join Taylor who was on my bed watching Peter Pan. The more we struggled with Matthew, the more her profound independence dwindled and the more starved for attention she seemed. I joined her on my bed and, as she smiled at me, I realized I needed to take the look of disappointment off my face. Even though Matt rarely looked at me, Taylor always did; and she sensed I was disappointed in her brother. I feebly returned the grin and joined her for the movie.

Prior to Matthew's assessment I had convinced CDS to set up an appointment with a local child designation psychologist. He would be the type of person who could give a diagnosis and could provide us with more information on the disorder, if that was indeed what Matthew had. When our appointment with the psychologist arrived, we were very anxious to attend. I had arranged for a sitter to come over and watch Taylor. Dallan came home early from work to accompany me.

At our visit we immediately sat down, and Matthew began to squirm in my arms. It was obvious he was nervous and wondering where we had brought him. Dr. Fink quickly presented several toys on the small table in front of us to help occupy some of his time. He presented Matt with a doll house filled with people and furniture. Matt slowly opened the front door and was excited to discover four identical cars within. They were all the same size and design, each a different, bright, primary color. He smiled and began lining them up across the table.

The doctor began reviewing our concerns, going over each of the things that Matthew seemed delayed in. He began asking many questions about Matthew's behavior and speech. In the past, the questions had been heart-wrenching and difficult to answer. But now we were so eager to find out what was going on, we raced on with explanations and offered our other harbored concerns. We talked about the spinning, banging, and other repetitive behavior. We talked about his language—or lack thereof. We discussed his hatred of change and strangers, and his lack of pretend-play and social skills. We spilled out our hearts.

The doctor also helped us realize other things about Matthew that were typical signs of autism that we had never noticed before. He flapped his hands when excited. He would hide under tables and chairs when nervous. He never pointed with his index finger to bring something to our attention. (I had forgotten how often our daughter had done this at his age.) Rubbing his ears and looking at things closely were other stimulatory behaviors he displayed. We realized more and more that he truly was in his own little world.

I felt an amazing the rush of emotions in that office. I was amazed and excited to find someone so knowledgeable of Developmental Disorders, but at the same time I was also terrified. Even though I had prayed and had been fasting all day that we would find out exactly what was going on, I deep-down hoped that our past assumptions were wrong. I could handle the embarrassment of telling people we were paranoid and over-protective. (Maybe somehow that meant I was a good mother.)

Dr. Fink next quietly watched Matthew. He tried to interact and involve himself in his play. People, puppets, puzzles—nothing would distract him from lining up the cars.

Dr. Fink then turned and asked us a question.

"In your minds, what do you think is wrong with your son?"

Dallan and I quickly glanced at each other mustering up a little courage. I stuttered and Dallan quickly cut me off,

"He has autism. I know it. "

I wish I had Dallan's strength. I was so worried about being labeled crazy. "I agree. I have done a lot of research..." I tried to back myself up, "and I really do think he has it."

We both froze in our chairs eagerly awaiting a response. He faintly smiled and said, "I think you are right. Matthew is autistic." And there it was!

I don't remember much else of the appointment with the psychiatrist. The visit that had seemed in slow motion was now flying so fast I could hardly keep up. I nodded as if I were absorbing it all, knowing it was going right through me. I sat there, finally allowing myself to contemplate what this meant for me and my family. I think the doctor mentioned it was too soon to tell the severity of Matthew's autism, that this would come in time after some therapy. What else he talked about I will never remember.

I refused to cry. I had to go home and face Taylor and act like everything was all right. I held it in and so did Dallan. Two hours later Taylor was in bed, Matthew was curled up on the couch, and Dallan was working on the computer. I lay down on the couch with my head in Matthew's small lap. He always loved it when I lay down, allowing him to twirl my hair in his small fingers. He and I had a silent arrangement; if he wouldn't eat it, I would indulge him and I would put up with the twirling and pulling.

As he wrapped his fingers in the short lengths of my hair, the crying finally came. It did not just arrive knocking at the door; the grief flowed in, knocking down the door and myself with it. I lay there not wanting ever to move or to have to look at my son again. I could not help but feel I had failed him. Whether this disorder was genetic or not, he was my son; and I felt as helpless as any mother can.

I spent many hours that night and weekend on the phone, mostly with my mother, who had been a wonderful source of help and comfort through all our difficulties. I felt sheepish after learning she had researched autism even more than I. She seemed to be knowledgeable about different treatments; and she was eager to help us get started on rescuing Matthew. She located the Autism Society of Utah where she lived, and she visited a local school with children who also were diagnosed with autism. She figured, "Maybe if I reach out and help here, someone will reach out and help you there."

I knew she wished she lived closer to help us with Matthew, but her desire and strength to help gave me comfort enough. I was grateful for our closeness and her constant support.

I slept that night with swollen eyes and a broken heart. How was I ever going to help my son get better? The next morning brought no comfort, only a sharp migraine. On the phone my mother and I wept again and again. I had never felt so hopeless before.

I also prayed. I knew my husband and my faith were the only things that would get me through this. Dallan was my strength, and my beliefs were my will to go on. I prayed for comfort; I prayed for peace. And most of all I prayed to make it through the day.

"Say Mom.""Mom. Mom. Mom. Mom. Mom."We went through this every day.

"Matthew, say Mom. It's not hard. Come on. Mom!"

"Ish, Ish, Icks Ack."

I swear he spoke German better than he did English. At least I got a response this time. His face was twisted, and he seemed to be telling me off as he wriggled free from my arms. We did get the occasional "Da da da da da da" out of him. It had no meaning. He just seemed to like repeating it once in a while.

"All right. That's it. No treat. Matthew, if you say Mom you can have a treat..." He walked away without looking back. I followed him and shoved a cookie in his face.

"Just look at me, Matty?"

He glanced at the cookie, which happened to be right in front of my face. His little fat fingers reached out, and I gave the cookie up.

"Good enough."

Some days I felt like I got through to him. Some days we made eye contact all the time, but other days, none at all. He chooses his time and his terms when he is willing to come into reality.

The following week Dallan and I returned for a second visit to the psychiatrist. We went over Matt's case and reported that in the last week nothing had changed—except for the increase in Matt's repetitive head-banging. The doctor again confirmed his diagnosis, made some notes, and asked us if we had any remaining questions. I mustered up some courage and tried to ask what was really in my heart.

"Are you really sure this is what Matthew has? I mean, I know he has it, but is there a chance we are wrong? I believe you, but um, I guess I have some friends who are doubting, and their doubts are very convincing. They don't seem to think Matt is so bad when they see him. I am just so confused about what to tell them. Matthew is frustrated, yes; but sometimes he seems so happy and fine," I pleaded.

"What do your friends expect? Do they want him to sit in a catatonic state swaying back and forth all day long? Matthew is autistic. He has lost all language skills, will not socialize with others, and has developed every typical behavior on the list. If they can't see that, then they don't understand what autism is."

He went on, "Do you think your son is autistic?"

"Yes." I reluctantly replied.

"Then let's stop worrying about if he has it, and start concentrating on how to help him live with it."

If only I had the doctor's courage. If only I had Dallan's strength. They were right. Matt was autistic, and I had to focus on helping him. I felt a deep sense of forgiveness for the misjudgment of my friends. My friends did not live with Matthew. They did not understand our pain and frustration. And deep-down I knew they meant well. I also felt shame. Through my anger and frustration I had wrongly judged them. I was so engulfed in my problem I didn't realize that they would never understand what I was going through, just like I would never understand some of their trials. Their disbelief was because they did not want to believe Matthew was different. Perhaps one day they would understand.

Mid-May soon arrived and we began preparing for Matthew's second birthday. Matthew's four-hour assessment came and went, and I began to prepare for our first IFSP (Individualized Family Service Plan). At this meeting I would find out what services we could receive and for how many hours we would receive state funding.

In the meantime I spent all my spare time researching what type of therapy would be most beneficial for Matthew. Once again it was up to me to decide: auditory integration, facilitated communication, play therapy, holding therapy, behavioral therapy. Which one was best? Being a firm believer in research, I looked for what was backed up by science and had some firm proof of success. Behavioral therapy seemed to have the most documented success. I came across a specific type called ABA. I was intrigued when I found the following:

Applied Behavioral Analysis is an intensive, structured teaching program. Lessons to be taught are broken down into their simplest elements. These elements are taught using repeated trials where the child is presented with a stimulus (like "do this" or "touch object" or "look at me"). Correct responses and behaviors are rewarded with LOTS of positive reinforcement. When incorrect responses occur, they are ignored; and appropriate responses are prompted and rewarded. Undesirable behaviors are approached in the same manner. At first, the child may be rewarded for doing something close to the desired response. Over time, as the child masters the lesson, expectations are raised and primary reinforcers (like bits of food) are replaced with social reinforcers (hugs, praise, etc.). As the child masters the skill and generalizes it, it becomes self-reinforcing.

Once simple skills like table readiness, imitation, attention and others are learned in this manner, they can be combined into more complex skills, like language, imitation, play skills, social interaction, and more. Since children within the autism spectrum vary enormously in their strengths and weaknesses, individualized lessons are developed to meet the particular needs of a given child.

A typical program consists of up to 40 hours per week of intensive one-on-one teaching on a year-round basis for two or more years. Teaching may be done by families, by professionals, or by volunteers guided by an expert consultant. Teaching usually begins in the child's home, but it may also begin in a school.

Research has documented recovery rates of 40 to 50 percent among children who started ABA between the ages of 2 and 5. There are many reports of significant improvements (but not recovery) in children who started at 7, 8, and later. Recovery in these studies was defined as children who attended school as "typical children" without support. In addition to the recovered children, an additional 40 percent of the children were mainstreamed with some support.

Most of the research-documented success involves children who had between 30 to 40 hours of ABA on a year-round basis for at least two years.

Although all children on the autistic spectrum are different, this therapy seemed to me to be what would most likely benefit Matthew. My desire to learn more grew and again I spent all waking hours researching ABA.

It was difficult to find time for both of the kids while doing all of my studying. I was spending more and more time researching. Soon everyone began feeling neglected. I was playing less with the children, and Dallan was lucky to get even a glance when he returned home from work.

"Hi, Nat. How was your day? How were the kids?" I looked up from my book. "Fine. Kids are fine."(Back to reading. Back to my crusade.)

That's it. I have to escape. I have to get out. I want out! I cannot do this any longer. I will not subject my family to living with a "ghostly" mother.

I stretched my arms and put my book down. My heart began to ache. I mean really ache. Sharp pains shot through my chest and my neck. What was going on? Is the pain in my head starting to spread?

I clasped my chest, pressing my hands firmly on my collar bones. I began breathing heavily and felt cold, then hot. Nothing brought me comfort. I just had to wait this out. All the while, Dallan was in the next room on the phone. He saw me pass the living room clutching my body.

"Honey, are you okay?"

Five minutes later I answered.

"Yeah, I am okay." I said, reappearing in the doorway. "Can you watch the kids while I run to the market? I will be right back."

"Yeah, okay, have fun." He smiled.

The pain had eased up and I wondered what was wrong with me. What was I doing to myself?I threw on a jacket and shoes and raced out to the car. The pain in my chest had mostly ceased, but it flickered back every few minutes.I walked slowly down each aisle. I felt foolish for coming here—only finding two or three things we needed at home. But where else would I have gone?

My mind raced as I continued to pace the aisles. Autism, autism, autism. My son has autism. Why am I not handling this by now? I finally walked to the check-out.

"How are you today?" the cashier asked.

"Fine, thanks, and you?" Did you know that my son has autism? That's right—autism. Oh, don't worry, he's fine. We're all fine.

I threw the bags in the trunk and returned home.

Please God, help me get through this. I have got to stop. But when? When will my mind be at ease? When will the research come to an end? When will my knowledge about autism be so complete that I stop making our small town library borrow books from Connecticut to Canada?

And what about my poor Taylor? Is our world full of autism right for her? Inside I have the desire to fight, to go on. But will Taylor survive this? Will she handle the chaos yet to come? Or will she grow up ashamed of her brother and her parents, who seem so different from the rest of the world?

And what about my marriage? Will it survive this? How can we take care of someone who might need our special attention for the rest of our lives? How will Dallan and I survive the constant needs and stress with this child?

A few days later my heart had seemed to calm. My prayers were fervent and pleading for guidance and I felt blessed with the assurance that I would be guided to find what was best for Matthew. Deep-down I knew that I would be able to withstand this great challenge as a mother. Somehow I would organize therapy for Matthew.

I spent the entire month of June visiting different special schools in the state. Five different ones were available, all within an hour's drive. I was constantly on the phone interviewing teachers and program directors, but the feeling of sending off my two-year-old overwhelmed me.

I tried to learn more about this Applied Behavioral Analysis and find out which of the schools offered it. I found one that seemed to inspire me: The May Center, north in Freeport. To my excitement, not only did they offer ABA at their school, they also offered it in our home. I immediately called Child Developmental Services, and yes! they would help us fund ABA therapy in our home!

For the first time in a long time we rejoiced! I had prayed and felt that if I pursued, this therapy would work out. Although we were still a long way from starting, we knew we had finally taken one step forward. It was a good thing, too, because Matthew was getting worse. He was not only banging and slapping his head more often, but he had started some new habits. As time slowly passed, his frustration increased; and he began pinching, scratching, and biting.

Heavenly Father, you have to help me. You have to help Matthew. We can't wait any longer. He needs your help. You have blessed me with the ability to care for him and the energy to fight for him. I have done all I can for him. He is in your hands.

Friday, June 21st, a miracle happened! I met the perfect match for Matthew. The May Center had called just a few days before—much earlier than I had expected—and surprised me with the news of an available therapist. Her name was Jan. She lived over an hour north from us, but was willing to make the daily trip.

I was amazed after the first few minutes they spent together. When Matthew met Jan, he immediately sensed her presence. He did not interact with her; but when she approached him, he continued playing quietly on the floor. Her quiet demeanor and gentle presence were not a threat to him so he allowed her to sit down right next to him. This to me was amazing. He rarely reacted this way with new people. We scheduled to begin our at-home ABA therapy the following Monday morning. Our fervent prayers had finally been answered.

For six months Jan drove to our home four days a week for a total of fifteen hours per week. Matthew also began receiving speech and occupational therapy as well. The ABA was very difficult in the beginning. Matthew spent most of the hours crying. Jan began with very simple tasks such as making eye contact, sitting in a chair, or playing with simple toys like shape-sorters and staking rings. He struggled, and so did the rest of us. But slowly we saw Matthew change. He tolerated the programs better, cried less, and began bonding with Jan. Just four months after we began, I wept as I watched him take Jan's hand and walk back to the therapy room. What a huge difference this behavior was, compared to the screaming and crying four months before.

After six months Matthew still had a long way to go, but we saw a much happier child. He had learned to request help from us by signing. His aggressive and self-injurious behaviors had almost diminished. He tolerated new people better and was interacting more with his family. Matthew still had not developed any language, so we began focusing on communicating in other ways. There were many more hills to climb, but we were finally heading up.

In November we began preparing Matthew for school. An opening at the May Center had been presented to us; and although I spent many hours praying and in tears wishing he didn't have to go, I knew it was the right decision for him. His therapy at home was extremely stressful, especially on our sweet Taylor. We knew he needed more, but it would be impossible to increase his hours at home. After much prayer, we knew we were choosing the best path for Matthew.

Just days before he was scheduled to begin, my small family knelt together in prayer. This time we didn't ask for guidance; we wanted to give thanks. We knew we had another challenge before us, but our previous experiences had made us stronger. We thanked our Father in Heaven for giving us Matthew and for giving us the courage to go on. This is where our journey begins.

As I look over my life, I constantly wonder how I was thrown into the world of autism. We are still only in the beginning of this foreign world, but through our struggle of discovering Matthew's disorder we seem to have somehow found peace. Our crusade has just begun, but every day I realize more and more that I do not need to know why. Perhaps that will be answered in the life to come. I love Matthew and that will keep me going for now. I will still struggle, and I will still have days that will seem more unbearable than any before. I still cry when I think of my small son who has never in his lifetime spoken the word, "Mom." Maybe he never will. But the importance of that task dwindles as I strive every day just to make sure his life is a happy one. We now understand our Matthew. Autism is not something he has, it is who he is. We will continue to fight the problems autism brings, to help him to learn to function in a "foreign world"; but we will never wish he were without it. Autism is who he is, and we love him.

Chapter Two

"To Taste the Bitter that We Might Know the Sweet "
Ayden, age 5
Ethan, age 4
Rowan, age 2
by Carly Johnson

Carly Johnson is an amazingly busy woman! In February of 2004, for Ayden's fifth birthday, she and Erik put on what turned into a huge "autism carnival" for the whole community. She has devoted many hours to raising autism awareness in her community. Ayden was diagnosed with severe food allergies, asthma and autism in the medium to mild range by age 2 years 8 months. Recently, Rowan was also diagnosed with autistic spectrum disorder.

I was the typical, rebellious teen. Erik and I started dating when I was 16 and he was 17. Two weeks after we began dating he told me he "intended to marry" me. I told him that was fine but that he would "never see me again" if he "ever tried to convert me."

I had grown up in an LDS family. We went to church on Sunday or else! I tested the "or else" too many times, and my parents finally gave up on me when I told them I was an atheist. It was the "in thing" among my crowd.

Erik was a bit off from the rest of the crowd. Erik looked a little like he was left over from the 70's. He always wore a gray, Levi jacket no matter the temperature. The jacket bore a button on the front that read, "Just visiting this planet." If you stuck around and talked to Erik awhile you would probably believe the button. In the pockets of his jacket he carried "everything." If anyone needed anything, he had it in his jacket pocket.

He was still very much a part of us, but he knew who he was and what he believed. Erik has always had an "old soul" feel to him. However, looking into his eyes, I could see the innocence and love for life of a new baby.

Almost everyone in our crowd was constantly in debate over anything, loved debating dearly, and would argue any point. Erik only stood up for what he believed, but he held his ground. He didn't argue for ego's sake, like most guys did; he taught what he believed, and he won on that ground constantly. Erik is very intelligent, but he used his intelligence without making a show.

I, on the other hand, was in and out of school. When I went at all I would only meet up with friends and leave again. By the last semester of my first year in high school I had failed all my classes except drama, and there I was only barely passing. Soon after Erik and I started dating, I was out of school for good.

I have no idea why I was so blessed to have caught Erik's attention. We were good friends for some time before he gave me a list of his "good and bad qualities." He wanted to be fair about the choice he was facing me with. He told me that he had a crush on me and wanted me to be able to make an accurate decision as to whether or not I could be with him. I was a "bad girl" at a school that was designated "drive-by high." Erik was the angel, and at any moment I expected him to realize how low he had stooped. I still can't figure out what Erik saw in me, but I'm glad he did. I don't know who else could have put up with me other than Erik.

After he made clear his intentions towards me, he told me we would have to wait about four years before we were married. He wanted to finish high school and go on a mission first. It took me 2 ½ years before I convinced him to stay home and marry me.

We were married in the Salt Lake City courthouse. If I had had my way, only Erik and I and the judge would have been there. I wanted it to be just between Erik and me: our stand of independence. I didn't want anyone to feel obligated to pay for anything having to do with our wedding. I tried to put our wedding rings on layaway to build up some credit, but I paid them off too quickly to accrue any. It seemed more important to me to enter a marriage with no debt than to establish credit. I didn't want to owe anything to anyone.

I didn't quite have the heart to outline it that way to my mother, however; and the mere suggestion of her not being at her daughter's wedding would not be tolerated. My parents and Erik's mother and stepfather were witnesses.

After two years of marriage, I finally convinced Erik that we should try to start a family. A very difficult two years later we were still trying. At that point I had to begin re-evaluating my life.

I have a very large family, and most of them are LDS. I was never truly able to escape going to Church because there was always a new baby's blessing or baptism or missionary farewell/homecoming to attend. It was about this time that I started noticing that the confusion and anguish over not yet having children seemed to disappear in the chapel. In fact I felt rather comforted there.

At the time I was at a horrible job that I hated so much I actually became physically ill. At one of those lowest moments on the job, I was just about ready to break down when I noticed that I had started to rock back and forth slightly with my arms cradled. At that moment the same calming feeling from the chapel came over me and in that instant I knew that I wasn't alone. As odd as it may sound I also knew that I had children waiting for me. I wasn't sure what that meant exactly but I knew they were there.

I tried to puzzle this out for some time. The next family event that took us to church again left me even more puzzled. I was so overwhelmed by the feelings I had there that I just cried through the whole hour. I was addicted to that feeling, and I tried to get more input about it.

I tried to get Erik to tell me about his testimony. He was pretty hesitant. I think he was thinking at the time that I was trying to bait him as an escape out of the marriage or something to that effect. He told me he did believe in the teachings of the church but not really a lot more than that.

After digesting that a bit, I told Erik that I felt that we did have children waiting for us. After some silence Erik assured me he felt the same way. We both felt there was more than one child waiting—possibly even three. One day it struck me that one of our children-to-be might be handicapped. Erik agreed it was likely. I asked him if knowing that possibility would change his mind about having children and was relieved to hear him answer that it wouldn't.

We eventually found the church building in our area and started attending sporadically. I always had that same feeling at church.

Yet, as time went on, we still had no children. I was lost and confused and finally decided to ask my dad for a father's blessing. The gist of the blessing was that if we did what we knew we needed to do, then the children would follow. I decided to receive my patriarchal blessing shortly after that. At the time it was being given, I got the feeling that I was being told, "Duh! I already told you this! Do what you know you need to do, and your blessings will follow."

Erik and I were sealed in the Salt Lake temple on our 5th wedding anniversary. Three months later we were pregnant.

Ayden was born 42 weeks later. The delivery was mostly uneventful. There were a few threats of a caesarean delivery due to meconium (first bowel movement in the womb/sign of stress to the baby) in the fluid. The baby's heartbeat was lost with each contraction and the cord was wrapped around the baby's throat. I was given a blessing, and I knew that everything would be as it should.

Once he had been born, the hospital staff rushed him off with Erik in tow. They needed to check his lungs to be sure that he hadn't swallowed any fluid. When they brought him back to me, he was wrapped in about ten blankets; and all that I could see of him were his eyes. The nurses said he was cold and to keep him covered. They had already counted his toes and fingers and pronounced him to be fine, so I kept him wrapped up, and I marveled over his eyes.

He was so alert! Those eyes showed so much intelligence. I just knew that with a father like Erik, he would have to be brilliant. I was so proud of him and so overwhelmed by all that we had been blessed with.

Reality struck hard and quickly though. I didn't sleep the whole time I was in the hospital. Ayden would try to nurse but only ended up sputtering and coughing up green liquid. They said he had swallowed the fluid in the womb and eventually they would have to pump his stomach. The nurse kept insisting that I wasn't nursing him correctly and tried to show me the correct way. I would try and try, but I could never get him to take in enough of the nipple to latch on.

Ayden never nursed correctly no matter how much I worked with him. But he seemed to enjoy nursing. In the first month he would wake up in the middle of the night and would nurse for five hours straight—with me crying because I was sore. If I tried to get him to stop and tried to comfort him in another way, he would scream until he was bright red and dripping with sweat; and the veins would pop out on his neck.

When Ayden did sleep he would laugh out loud. Two weeks after we brought him home, he would smile while he was awake! He could always, from birth, hold his head steady and within a few days after birth he bore all his weight on his legs and was doing the reflex "stepping" motion.

Ayden had to be in motion at all times. He wanted to be held but you couldn't sit down with him. He loved his swing. It was one of the very few ways he would fall asleep; but if you even thought about turning it off once he was sound asleep, he would wake right up.

He would fall asleep sometimes while nursing. I remember once seeing a commercial for some sort of baby product. The mommy was nursing the infant, and they were gazing into each others' eyes and cooing at each other. I remember laughing and thinking how stereotypical that was. Babies don't gaze at their mothers like that! I don't remember noticing that Ayden was specifically avoiding eye contact, but I wasn't really watching for anything like that at the time.

The only other way I could get Ayden to fall asleep was to rock him. He wouldn't have anything to do with gentle rocking back and forth though; it had to be fairly frantic. Even then he would scratch at his face to keep himself awake. But it would work if you held his arms (tightly, because he had amazing strength for an infant) down against his body.

We had to start him on cereal fairly early because he wasn't gaining enough weight. Once we started introducing solids, we discovered quickly that he was allergic to anything dairy. We couldn't even let anyone give him a kiss after drinking milk or it would leave a lip-shaped welt on him! If he ingested milk, he welted up all over—especially his eyes—and he would throw up and have some difficulty breathing. The welts would take days to go away completely. I brought pictures to his doctor who just said to give him soy formula or juice in his cereal; and that was the end of the discussion.

Erik got a job offer that would move us out of Utah and into Washington. When we went for the job interview, I knew it felt right and that we had to make the move. It was a hard thing to do because all of my family—and most of Erik's family—lived in Utah. But we did what we knew we needed to do. The same day when we found out that Erik was offered the job, we also found out I was pregnant again.

Ayden developed very quickly physically. The stepping reflex quickly turned to a fast-paced run and you had to struggle to keep holding his hands to keep up with him. He took his first steps alone by the time he was seven months old and was fully running by himself by the time he was nine months. Shortly after that he even learned to slow down to a walk. I was sure this was a sign of a genius child.

But starting a bit before Ayden turned one, he was sick all the time. He seemed always to have a flu bug or a cough; it never seemed to get better. At one point I realized that it was beyond flu. I kept taking him back to the doctor or calling the nurse, and they would say just to give him a while longer to get better. I figured they knew what they were talking about. Sometimes he would get better for a while, too. But at one point he was throwing up two to three times a day for about three weeks.

One morning I was feeding him some infant, mixed cereal, and he threw up again—only this time the vomit was streaked with blood.

I called for Erik to help me because I wasn't sure what to do. He didn't seem bothered by what I was pointing out to him. He insisted that it was probably some strawberries that had gone undigested from the lunch Ayden had eaten the day before. I was sure it was blood and was understandably upset by it. We called his doctor and took in a sample to them to be tested. It was blood.

I explained to them how long this had been going on, and the doctor said that it wasn't anything serious and that he most likely just ruptured a vein in his throat with the velocity of regurgitating. I remember being concerned that it was something worse than what he was describing— maybe something wrong with his stomach—and I asked if this was a possibility. The doctor "yelled" at me, saying that he was the one with the medical degree and that I shouldn't question him. I interrupted his shouting to apologize and tell him that I was just concerned for my son and that I wanted to be certain to understand what was happening.

Due to the length of time that Ayden had been sick, the doctors decided to do a few tests anyway. They took a urine sample, but it somehow got contaminated. They had to take a clean sample using a catheter. I had to help hold him down on the table while he screamed and cried like I had never heard him do before; and Ayden was the king of tantrums. We couldn't get him to sit on anything similar to a doctor's table after that for about six months (getting pictures taken was out of the question). They also did a reflux test and found a slight tendency but nothing that would cause him the problems he had been having.

Eventually they decided to send us to an allergist. Ayden's pediatrician had told us that we should try giving Ayden cheese or yogurt, saying that he might be able to eat that even though he had such severe reactions to every other dairy product. We tried giving him the smallest bit of cheese, and he had a huge reaction. I was glad to be able to talk to a specialist about the matter.

The allergist decided to do a scratch test. "Great, more traumatic tests," I thought. They tested him for all the basic allergens. Ayden turned out to be allergic to dairy, almonds, peanuts, eggs, and wheat. They all made sense to us except for the wheat, which showed up as the least of his allergens anyway.

We had considered all along that his problems very well could be allergy-related but could see no patterns. Egg was one that had really tripped us up because—when cooked in baked goods—sometimes the egg protein will break down enough that it is unidentifiable to the body as egg. So he would eat corn dogs just fine…until that third one where it wasn't broken down enough in baking.

We changed his diet, and he improved immediately. We were given directions on medications and what to watch for in case of an emergency. We learned that he had been having anaphylactic reactions. We took him off wheat (just in case) for three weeks and put him back on because he didn't seem to have any physical rejection of it. The doctor figured it would be fine for him to have it again. His being able to have wheat again was good because it was hard enough feeding this kid! But eventually he did make it to his first birthday. I don't know how he survived all the experimentation.

That wasn't the end of it though. Occasionally, he would still get the cough. He would cough and cough until he threw up. Or he would have a tantrum and cough and cough until he got sick. Then it started getting worse; he would cough and not throw up and not get better. It sounded similar to the breathing problems he had if he had eaten food he was allergic to, but we didn't see how that was possible.

At one point Erik took him to the emergency room for this problem, and they had him breathe from a machine called a nebulizer. It turned the liquid medication they put in it into a steam so that Ayden could breathe it in directly to the source of the problem; it helped him right away.

The next time Ayden reacted that way, we took him to his pediatrician's office again. We explained to them what happened at the ER visit, and they asked if we had been given a nebulizer to take home. Ayden was nebulized in the office, and we were sent home with a nebulizer of our own. After a lot of searching on our own, we figured out that Ayden had asthma and that was what was causing all the non-food, allergic reactions. Ayden was allergic to dust mites as well.

After a lot of education on subjects we knew nothing about, we were finally sailing again. Ayden was a bit behind in his language skills but after all that commotion, could you blame him?

When Ayden was about 16 months old, his baby brother Ethan was born. Ethan was very interactive. He looked straight at me within a few hours after he was born and cooed and stared at me, right in the eyes! That seemed odd to me, because Ayden had never done that. It almost seemed wrong to me to have a baby do that.

Ethan adored Ayden right from the start. At first he would just follow him with his eyes whenever Ayden came into his line of vision. A few months later, Ethan would smile and laugh and get so excited to see him. But from the day we brought Ethan home Ayden didn't really seem to notice Ethan. He never did more than glance at Ethan and that seemed to be only to make sure that Ethan didn't have anything he might want.

We took Ayden in for his 18-month check up. We couldn't get in with his regular doctor so we saw the nurse practitioner. She was a bit concerned about his language skills. Ayden only had about 20 words at that time. He seemed to pick up new words all the time but we never really heard the old ones again, so it was difficult to count exactly. The nurse suggested we have an evaluation done by a speech therapist, but she had to get Ayden's doctor's approval first. His doctor denied the request, wanting to wait until Ayden turned two—in hopes we would see some improvement by that time.

At his two-year-old check-up he had learned a few more new words, so she was encouraged. They wanted to wait until he turned three to see if he had caught up by then. I had a hard time waiting until he was two and was really starting to worry. Yes, he had learned some new words but he hadn't kept the old ones again. He was way behind other children his age, and the doctor wanted to put it off for another whole year?

One night I received an e-mail telling me all about the typical development of a 26-month-old. I had been receiving them every month of Ayden's life, something I had signed up for while I was pregnant with him. But this one had a link to an article entitled "When to see a speech therapist." That of course caught my attention, and I went to it right away. There was a list of warning signs to watch for—maybe thirteen different warnings. Ayden had all the signs except for one or two.

I was pretty frantic at that point. It had only been two months since Ayden's last appointment when the doctor had told me to wait and see, but I couldn't wait after seeing that article. I called the doctor's office and talked to the nurse to explain what I had just read and why I was worried. She said she would be concerned as well and made an appointment for us to get in to see the doctor again right away. We explained our concerns again to the doctor, and she referred us to get a developmental evaluation.

This was done by a "special needs 0-3" school. There was a team of four or five people, all asking us questions about Ayden and trying to get Ayden to do different things with them. They left us for a bit and came back with their results. Ayden was a year delayed in his speech. He was also delayed in his social skills and slightly in his physical skills (but that was mostly due to his not being able to take direction well).

I was pretty upset by it all. My son had been behind for so long, and I hadn't even helped him when I knew there was a problem. Instead I had listened to the doctor and let it go for six months longer than it should have. Now he would probably have to work hard for several years to catch up, so he wouldn't be so behind when he started kindergarten. Behind a full year in speech!!! That was half his life at that point!

The evaluation team suggested that he start school there, and they would work with him to help him catch up. They wanted us to go to have a "secondary evaluation" done. They also suggested that we go to a private speech therapist, and they gave us a list of names. Written in on the side of the list they handed us was Jen's name! I knew her! Her name had been mentioned just the day before when I had been visiting teaching. She was in our ward. I told the team that I knew her and that I wanted to enlist her help; it was the only thing that was familiar to me in this whole mess. They told me that they had just found out about her and had written her name on the list the day before. To me the window had opened for us when the door closed. I was so happy to see a light at the end of the tunnel, I had to struggle not to cry. I called Jen that night!

Jen was a full-time mom and a part-time speech therapist. She was only working two days a week, and only for a few hours on those days, but she was able to work us in. When I thought back about the day before the evaluation, I realized that everyone I had talked to that day had mentioned Jen's name for some reason or other. I had been meaning to ask her name because I had forgotten it. I had heard she was a speech pathologist and meant to call her to get her opinion regarding Ayden. I didn't even have to ask because everyone we saw while visiting teaching was talking about Jen. I think that Heavenly Father knows how dense I can be about names and was really trying to drill it in. It worked! As soon as I saw her name, I knew that no matter what happened it was going to be okay. How could it not be when we were looked after that well?

The next day I called to make the secondary evaluation with the neurologist that the speech therapists had suggested. The receptionist seemed a bit confused and asked "Is this for an evaluation to determine autism? That is all this office does." I was struck dumb. My eyes started welling up and my voice was shaking. "No one on the evaluation team had mentioned autism to me, they just suggested we get a secondary evaluation done, and they suggested this doctor." She informed me that it had to be for an autism evaluation in that case, and she proceeded to ask me a huge list of questions about Ayden. I answered the best I could as I tried to piece it all together for myself.

Autism! The only time that word had been mentioned at the evaluation was when I had said it regarding one of Ayden's behaviors. My friend had associated that behavior with a child she had met with autism, and so I mentioned that so that I could be reassured, laughed at even. No one really said much about it; in retrospect I should have taken that as a clue. I had been worried about there being more to it than just a speech delay because he was so significantly behind; but Erik had reassured me, and the doctor only sent us to the evaluation because of my insane worrying.... right? When my friend had even mentioned the "A word" in the same paragraph as Ayden, I became really angry that she would even remotely associate the two.

"No, no, you've got it all wrong. My son doesn't have autism. This is just a clear- cut case of an overly-worried, maybe even over-imaginative, first-time mom," I wanted to scream, as the receptionist rambled on about there being a three month waiting list and how she was going to send out some papers for me to fill out in the meantime.

In truth, I really had no idea what autism was. Rain Man was closest thing I could relate to in my knowledge on the subject. Rain Man seemed a far cry from my son. But suddenly my head was swarming with words like "eye contact," "social skills," "pretend play," "repetitive behaviors," and "appropriate toy play." Was I really supposed to have watched for all these things in my child? Does every mother know to watch for these things, and I was the only one not informed? I knew Ayden was different, but he had been sick and had all these other problems. I figured he was just much cleverer than the other children that wanted to do such silly things. I guess I had attributed it all to his personality. It wasn't as if his father and I were the norm.

While we waited for the neurologist's appointment, we started school and speech therapy. Ethan had a hard time watching Ayden get to play with all the cool toys, so I eventually enrolled him in the class as a role model student. He did very well in his role. Ethan had already started talking, and his vocabulary had surpassed Ayden's. Ethan would start a conversation with anyone in the class. You couldn't always understand him, but you could catch a word here and there. We were happy to see he was still trying to engage others in conversation, even though he had given up on getting Ayden to talk with him.

I soon discovered that there was a mothers' group that met during the class hours once a week. This was an amazing experience for me. Here, I was able to find out that I wasn't alone. I found I wasn't just a horrible mother who had caused all of these problems to happen to Ayden because of my lack of skill. I also found out a bit more about what was to come, what to expect next with him, and how to help him out. Plus I think I even helped other people to gain some understanding as well.

Since I grew up in Utah and lived there my entire life, it was a new experience to talk with people who didn't have that Utah language down. (Not to say that everyone in Utah is LDS, but there is such a majority there that everyone at least knows what a "ward" is.) I fumbled over terms like that here, and people would look at me like I was insane. "Ward?" they would say, backing up a bit, as if I had just come from a "psycho ward."

One time I was talking with a mother who had a child in Ayden's class. She was Catholic and had made a promise to God that she would dedicate her first son to Him. She said she would signify this by naming him Sebastian after Saint Sebastian. When her first son was born he had some brain damage and had physical and mental disabilities. She didn't feel it would be proper to dedicate this son to the Lord because he wouldn't ever be able to enter the priesthood. She said that for this reason she named her first son after Saint Nicholas and her second son was named Sebastian.

I was trying to comfort her by telling her that her son had most likely already been dedicated to the Lord in a lot of other ways. I tried to explain to her a non-doctrinal belief that I had heard several times, regarding a Down's syndrome child that had received his patriarchal blessing. In his blessing he was told that he had been given Down's syndrome to protect him from the Adversary. This was said to have been done because he was one of the angels to escort Lucifer out of heaven in the pre-existence.

"Pre-existence? What is that?"

My mouth dropped! I had no idea that people could grow up not knowing where they had come from. I tried to explain to her; but I was totally dumbstruck so I did it poorly. I told her that the Bible talked about the pre-existence in some places and that I would look them up for her and get back to her.

I went immediately to my nearest LDS book store, bought her a Book of Mormon, took it home, and Erik and I found all the scriptures having anything to do with the pre-existence and highlighted them. We then cross-referenced them with scriptures in the Bible and wrote all those down for her. I wrote an inscription trying to explain better the story I had fumbled so badly before. And I gave her a picture of Jesus holding a child; the picture was inscribed at the bottom, "Precious in His eyes."

I gave these items to her, and the next time I saw her she thanked me and told me my gift had really touched her. She said that she understood the principles and felt really good about them. "I believe what you told me and it brings me comfort," she said. Not only did I bring her comfort but I felt like I "planted a really beautiful seed" in her. I didn't push anything on her; but I did continue to bring her different LDS pictures, which she loved and framed and hung up all over her house. I love to imagine the missionaries coming to visit her some day and being encouraged by all those pictures.

The "0-3 school" was such a good experience for us. The only thing that I think we needed more was Jen. At enrichment night, I had taken a "Baby Sign" class which Jen had taught, and I had already been implementing that method. But once Jen became our speech therapist, she did so much for our family. Take note that I didn't say she became Ayden's speech therapist. She was ours. She taught Ayden, yes; but she also taught us what we could do to help Ayden. She taught us—plus she was there for all my concerns and could help to offer solutions and insights.

But one of the things I appreciate so much about Jen was the insight she dared give us when no one else would. I kept getting the feeling that everyone working with Ayden knew what his diagnosis would be, but they wouldn't confront me about it. They would say what options would be available to him if he were diagnosed with autism. Then they would scuttle back and say that he might be diagnosed to be perfectly normal and that would be even better. They would say just enough to let me know that they knew something was different, but they wouldn't affirm any of it. It was driving me mad—mainly because by this time I had read up on autism as much as I could. Everything I found out about it led me to believe that my son had autism. But I had no one I could discuss our problem with, and I felt guilty for even thinking that autism could be Ayden's difficulty.

When I tried to discuss Ayden's problems with Erik, he would tell me I was just worrying too much. He just kept telling me he thought Ayden was behind because of all his other problems. Or (Erik would say) that Ayden had concentrated too much on walking early and on climbing and all the physical stuff. Now we had to teach him to expand his vocabulary. He thought social skills would come after Ayden's vocabulary improved.

I would show Erik some information on autism, and he could see how perfectly it described Ayden; but then Erik would brush it aside because he wanted to wait to see how Ayden was diagnosed before jumping to any conclusions. Besides, Erik didn't understand the necessity of having a label placed on his son anyway.

Six months later we finally were able to get an appointment with the neurologist. About a week before we were supposed to go in to be evaluated, Jen took me aside after Ayden's speech therapy. "I just wanted to tell you before you go in," she said, "Ayden is likely to be diagnosed somewhere in the autistic spectrum. I'm not positive about this, but I'm fairly certain. The only reason that I want you to know this is because I want you to deal with the possibility now, before you go in to get the diagnosis from the doctor. I want you guys to deal with the grief that it can cause now, so that you can be aware of what happens at Ayden's appointment. I want you to be able to ask the things you need to ask and say the things you need to say instead of dealing with grief and being too overwhelmed by it all at that time."

I went home and told Erik what she had said. It was probably one of the best pieces of advice that we could have been given. By the time the evaluation was over and we went in to get the diagnosis, Erik and I had both read up enough and figured that Ayden was somewhere in the middle of that autistic umbrella. The neurologist diagnosed Ayden as having autistic spectrum disorder in the medium to mild range. The doctor told us that due to Ayden's age, the diagnosis of autism was hard to document, so the diagnosis could possibly change when he got older. Ayden, however, did have some fairly classic symptoms.

I had dealt with a lot of the grieving process before the diagnosis. Erik had come to terms with it a bit, but it wasn't until the hard diagnosis that he dealt with the grief. When I thought about the dreams I had about being a mother, they were mostly about being able to talk with my children and teach them by explaining things to them. My main question for the doctor was if Ayden would ever be able to talk. Of course the specialists couldn't tell me that for sure. They did give some hope of Ayden's becoming more verbal because he used some words now, "but there are just no guarantees."

It was about this time that we found out we were pregnant again. We were still feeling so overwhelmed with our other two children, and we were being very careful to postpone pregnancy. With Ethan we had tried to conceive so early only because it had taken so long to get pregnant with

Ayden that we figured we might have to wait a while.. This time we didn't even try to conceive, and surprise! Right after Ayden's diagnosis, another pregnancy was the last thing I wanted to deal with. We announced the forthcoming birth, but I guess we seemed less than enthusiastic about it. One of the ladies at Ayden's "0-3 school" told me that she would be willing to adopt the baby if we couldn't accept it at this time. I tried to explain to her how important my kids are to me and that there really wasn't any way I could ever deal with giving one away. "I am excited about this baby," I told her. "It's just that it's an overwhelming thing to think about at a time when you find out your oldest child has autism. I just don't think I will be able to think about the pregnancy until I deal with the autism issue. But I do fully understand the gift that our children are to us. We were told that we wouldn't be able to have children, and now we are working on our third!" The only way to explain my mixed feelings and emotions to anyone was to bear them my testimony of this gospel.

Thinking about my testimony made me realize how much of a gift life is, how much of a gift every one of these children are. I think that one of the reasons our Heavenly Father wanted to wait until Erik and I were sealed to send us Ayden was that he wanted us to realize fully the gift we were being given. He knew that we would need the help that the gospel brings and the blessings that come with being sealed in order to get us through this difficult time. Ayden has taught us a lot about ourselves, a lot about some of our weakest spots, but a lot about good, too.

Ethan has never ceased to be a blessing to our family either. He has had an unfailing love for Ayden from the day he was born. When he was six months old, Ethan took his first steps trying to run after Ayden! Ethan taught us so much about what we should be looking for Ayden to be doing. Ethan's typical development helped us to see that there was actually a problem with Ayden. Otherwise, we probably wouldn't have had any concerns for Ayden at all. Ethan keeps Ayden social and engaged, when Erik and I are too tired and too worn down to do it.

We were excited about another sibling for these boys because we wanted Ayden to see what typical social behavior would be like. We were excited for Ethan to have a playmate that played with him willingly—without having to be chased down every few seconds. We were scared for us, having these kids so close in age, but excited for them, hoping that the minimal age difference would allow them to be closer friends. We were truly excited and feeling very blessed about this new addition to our family; but soon after Ayden's diagnosis, we had very little time to think about it.

The neurologist insisted that Ayden be in a minimum of 25 hours of therapy a week. So, in addition to the time Ayden spent in the classroom at his "0-3 school," he also attended an autism-specific class there. We doubled his speech therapy time with Jen, enrolled him in music therapy, and put our names on waiting lists for an occupational therapist and for the University of Washington autism center program. We were told that there would be about six months' wait for the U of W program.

I remember feeling like such a failure in the first few months after the diagnosis. Ayden had only about half the hours that the doctor had said were the minimum. I broke down one night and cried and cried until I found myself on my knees begging my Father for help. After we had our names on the list for about six weeks, the U of W called us to tell us they had an opening. I felt like I was cheating because I didn't tell them we hadn't waited the specified time. (I didn't dare breathe a word of it because I was so excited to get Ayden started.)

It was a half-hour drive to the "0-3 school" and half an hour back. We would have to go out there sometimes twice a day. Ethan learned to take naps while we drove or else he wouldn't have had any naps at all. I refused to give Ayden naps anymore, because when he napped he would not sleep at night. I had to choose my battles with Ayden and nap time just wasn't worth it. This was a very hard time for me anyway. I lost a lot of weight because the pregnancy made me so sick and because I was running all the time. (By the end of this pregnancy I had gained a total of only two pounds.) I felt so overwhelmed by all the difficulties. How could a two-and-a-half-year-old keep up this pace? He did though, and he seemed to love every minute of it. He did not walk but ran to class and never looked back to check up on me. Some of his behaviors even seemed to lessen in severity. He was getting what he needed there.

At the time I hadn't thought about how fortunate we were to have insurance, but in retrospect I realize how lucky we were. All of Ayden's therapies were being covered by Erik's insurance that he received at work. Not only did they cover these therapies, but they were the only company in the country that covered ABA therapy. The realization of why the Spirit led us away from our families to this particular place became very obvious at that point. This was the best place we could have possibly been to get Ayden the help he needed.

My therapy came in the form of the mothers' group at the "0-3 school." It was so good to go there each week; I could hardly wait. I would make mental lists of everything I wanted to discuss with the other mothers. I'm sure I could have looked up the information myself on the questions I had—and in fact I did on a lot of them—but nothing beat the understanding that I got from actual parents having problems similar to mine. I don't think I sought out solutions as much as the feeling of not being alone.

Often I felt isolation in my ward. Don't get me wrong; I think we have one of the closest-knit wards there is. There is a toddler group in our ward where the mothers with toddlers meet once a week to do different activities. They have time to be with other adults that way. We tried to attend this group several times, but Ayden is too overwhelmed by wide open spaces. He has no fear of getting lost, so he bolts (as soon as he can squirm away from me). Ethan thinks it's a game, so he bolts in the opposite direction. These outings became way too exhausting for me, and I didn't end up going to very many for that reason. I didn't get the grown-up talk that I needed while I chased the boys anyway.

The major thing that made me feel isolated in our ward, however, was when all the ladies met for a monthly scrapbooking party. It was girls' night out, and we all would meet at someone's house and work on whatever projects we needed to get finished. We would stay up into the wee hours of the morning, while chatting about our husbands and children. I thought this sounded like a fantastic opportunity because I had so many projects I was working on for Ayden's therapies.

However, after Ayden was diagnosed, my projects seemed more and more peculiar; and no one understood or identified at all with the stories I had about my kids. I'm not normally a quiet person in situations like this, but I found myself quiet more and more at these parties. Eventually, I would go home crying. I couldn't identify with a typically-developing family anymore. The realization hit me that we not only had a special needs child, but we were also a special needs family. Autism affected every member of our family even though it was only Ayden with the diagnosis.

We doubled Ayden's hours when we started the ABA-style (Applied Behavioral Analysis) home therapy through the U of W. He couldn't have been happier. He was doing so well with his various therapies, too. In school they started him on PECS (Picture Exchange Communication System). He would give us pictures of things to tell us what he wanted. From this, I think, he started to get an understanding of what communication was for.

We had been trying to teach him some basic sign language for a year; but after he was introduced to PECS he actually started signing along with the pictures! His eye contact was improving by leaps and bounds. Ethan even taught Ayden to point to things that he wanted! The methods were all going along so smoothly—until he turned three.

Ayden's third birthday came four short months after his diagnosis. We had an IEP (Individual Education Plan) for him that was a mess. I think they must have evaluated someone else's child to come up with the goals that they did for Ayden. None of the goals made sense to me, but I couldn't get the school district to work with us on it. Though Ayden seemed to love the classroom, he was starting all sorts of odd behaviors and was regressing from all the progress he had already made.

Ayden was starting preschool in a classroom with five or six children and a teacher with two teacher's aides. All the children in his class had autistic tendencies or had an autism diagnosis. However, Ayden's food allergies made quite a commotion, and the school nurse and teachers were very apprehensive about Ayden's being there.

They delayed his getting into the class so that they could instruct the teachers how to administer Benadryl and the EpiPen in case of an emergency. We also had to get a lot of papers signed from Ayden's doctor telling them what he could and couldn't have to eat. They wanted to know exactly what he was allergic to and what signs to watch for.

We tried to tell them that since Ayden had started on a daily asthma medication his food allergy reactions were much less severe and typically only required a small dose of Benadryl. I guess having all the precautions in place is good; but it seems so odd that we, as Ayden's parents, weren't allowed to teach anyone about the precautionary measures to take with our son. It was odd, too, that they wouldn't take our word regarding his allergies. It seemed to me that this was the beginning of really losing my son.

It took several months for Ayden to get to a point where he regained some of the skills he had lost in that transition. He actually started to learn again. Then a few short months later he was out of school for the summer. His home therapist got a new job in another state, plus, we had a new baby brother at home. Ayden started pulling his hair out by the handfuls, and he destroyed everything he could get his hands on. He even tore baseboard molding off the walls.

After Ayden started school with the school district, I really started feeling that I didn't know what was going on with him anymore. I tried to communicate with his teacher at every opportunity and even went in to observe the class, but I just didn't have that daily feedback that I had before.

Before, during, and after the pregnancy, I also lost track a lot with his ABA and other therapies. At times, I felt that I never got to spend any time with Ayden because of his therapies. I felt like I was constantly fighting just to find out what was going on with him. Now that he is in a classroom, his teacher never has the time to keep me updated. His therapies seem to go on just fine—even if I am out of the loop. The general reports are that he is doing well. I am struggling to stay well informed again, so I can advocate for my son and communicate the needs that he can't express for himself. It's not an easy task with two other children; but they buoy me up and keep me going, too.

During Ayden's appointments, most of his therapists must think I am crazy to wait around with such small children in tow; but for now being there keeps me "in the loop." Plus, I get more one-on-one time (so to speak) with Ayden's two brothers during these times. I like to think that my spending time with them strengthens them, so they can be stronger for Ayden. Our lives, now, are full of ups and downs; they are used to that. It's amazing how much you can teach and learn during quiet time in a waiting room.

I thought for a while that I was losing my mind. I can never seem to remember anything anymore. I lock my keys in the car constantly now. However, it normally works out okay because I also, fairly consistently, forget to lock at least one door. I am doing things like that so often that I have really started to worry about myself. Does Alzheimer's strike at age 28? But then I realized one day that when your kids force you to run faster than you have strength, confusion is bound to happen. I am hopeful that by the time the baby has his first birthday I will have recovered a bit.

I have the feeling that, to some extent, life will always be this roller coaster. It has been only one year since Ayden was diagnosed. In some ways the year has gone by so fast, but in other ways time seems to have dragged out over twenty years. Ayden will be four soon. Though he is now able to label things when asked, he still doesn't have much spontaneous language. Ayden has made a lot of improvements and almost seems to be a different boy to our families (when we get a chance to visit with them). A comparison with kids that are Ayden's age now, though, is very difficult. As excited as we are that we are now having conversations with Ethan, we have difficulty seeing him pass Ayden in this area.

Erik has traded in that fresh look on life for a tired and worn one. He is a loving father and works so hard; then he comes home and works harder. But he is stronger for this effort. I have never been an easy person to get along with, but Erik has made it through all our struggles to even greater ones, and has fared all the better for it. I am so proud of him. Erik is my strength, my confidant, my love.

I have so many fears for Ethan and for my youngest, Rowan.—not so much that they might someday show signs of autism (though that is never far from my mind) but that they will fare poorly because of all this stress. I know that they will be obliged to become stronger as well. They will have to gain a deeper understanding of people and be less likely to judge. I am excited to see them grow into young men because I know I will be proud of them, but I can't help but have this deep sorrow for them for all that they will be required go through along the way. I am sure that it is just a taste of what our Heavenly Father goes through from sending us to this life.

I am still so uncertain what the future holds for us and for Ayden. I had always hoped that I could make up for keeping Erik from his mission some day. I figured that we would have the chance for the two of us to go on a mission after the kids grew up and moved out. The realization has hit me that this dream might not be a possibility now.

Another big realization hit me when I was vacationing back in Salt Lake last Christmas. My sister and her family were staying with my parents at the time that we came to stay with them for our visit. My sister has three small children, so we had to struggle to try to keep Ayden away from the foods he couldn't have. We ended up giving Ayden medicine to counteract his food reactions every day we stayed with them.

I was so frustrated at one point and was complaining to my mother. "One day he will be old enough to understand what he can and can't eat," she consoled. "No Mom," I retorted, "I'm not sure that he will ever understand that. We can't even get him to take direction enough to use an inhaler for his asthma, and I'm not sure that he will ever even be able to tell us that he is having an asthma attack. There are no guarantees for us that Ayden will ever gain that understanding." After I said that, I realized just how true it was and how hard it will be if that is what the future holds.

These thoughts came on me suddenly, and there is a bit of grieving that comes back with each of these realizations. But slowly, when these thoughts come to me, I have started to wonder instead what the Lord will open up for us and what I need to learn from this experience. At times like that, I'll look back and remember how independent I used to be. One of my biggest struggles now is accepting help when I need it.

Another factor I am struggling to overcome is all the well-meaning people who try to tell me that they can relate to my situation. Even my bishop, soon after I had Rowan, told me that they had their first three children similarly spaced, so they completely understood how difficult that could be. I have numerous relatives telling me funny stories meant as antidotes to my current problems. I know they are trying to help, but I really have to struggle not to bite their heads off at times. I just want to explain to them that they come from a typically-developing family and that they have no idea what I am going through.

Even if their children are similarly spaced to mine, I'm sure their oldest child was a lot more helpful or could at least follow some simple instructions. At the very least he could stop doing something he knows he shouldn't be doing (when you can do nothing more than scream at him because you are knee deep in another problem). Ethan can help me do small things, like getting a diaper, and I know that when he is Ayden's age he will be a huge help to me. But Ayden, developmentally, is far behind Ethan in this respect. It's almost like having a two-year-old, an 18-month old (with some horribly destructive habits) and a three-month-old.

I am learning, very slowly, to bite my tongue whenever I hear someone say they understand what we are going through. I put on my most grateful smile, and then I try to tune out every word. I used to deflect everything they told me as politely as I could, but I fear that my effort never went over very well. I'm not very good at being the passive type in things that are so near my nerves. I'm trying.

I am still constantly searching for answers to so many questions. I haven't ever asked, "Why has the Lord done this to me?" like so many people do in this kind of situation. I will never understand, however, what the Lord sees in someone like me, who was once a rebellious teen, who still hasn't even finished high school, and who has failed in so many other avenues of life. Why would He think that I could handle such a precious gift as Ayden? I know I am a daughter of my Heavenly Father, and I love Him as He does me. I know He knows me better than I know myself, and I pray that I can live up to His expectations. Failure is not a choice when it comes to my family.

Ayden tries at every turn to teach us patience. I do better with it now than I did, and Erik is learning what it feels like to lose his patience. I have learned to trust my instincts more. I have learned that "instinct" is frequently the Spirit's speaking to you. I have learned the strength that can come from dealing with a handicap.

I know that our Father loves us regardless of creed. I see the guidance of the Spirit and the love of family, which is taught to LDS families, so strong in other families that have special needs children. I think their children teach them more of the gospel than they realize. Just as Ayden has been a strength and a teacher in our lives. I have learned from him not to depend on words so much to understand the people I love. I have learned that conversation isn't necessary to learn about someone enough to love them. I see the love he has for others unconditionally and I can see that Ayden is bringing new understandings to everyone around him.

My greatest fears have always been of the unknown. I have no idea what we might be able to expect of Ayden. I am unsure how this will affect his brothers. I am no longer positive of what Erik and my future together might hold. But I know that, even when I completely turned my back on the Lord, he never gave up on me. He knows my path better than I do, and if I trust in Him everything will be as it should.

Chapter Three

Xander, age 5
Ben, age 3
Amy Umble

For as long as I can remember, I have had a strong faith in Heavenly Father that has never let me down. Until I found out that my younger son had autism. For a long time after Ben was diagnosed, I remained in a fog of bitterness and despair that separated me from Heavenly Father.

I had brought Ben to the pediatrician when he was two and a half, because he had stopped talking. I was desperate, and I begged the doctor to find something, anything physically wrong with Ben. Anything that would cause him to stop speaking, except for the one thing I feared most: that he, like his older brother, was autistic.

The doctor checked him over and ran tests. She was almost as eager as I was to find something else, but at the end, she called me into the office and shook her head. "I think you'd better call the autism specialists," she told me regretfully. And then she looked at me and asked, "Are you going to be okay?"

I couldn't answer her; I just burst into tears. There was no way, I thought numbly, no way Heavenly Father would do this to me.

I had been faithful and righteous, I felt. When the doctors diagnosed Xander, my older son, with autism, I hadn't been overly upset. While it wasn't something I would have chosen, I knew that Heavenly Father had a plan for us as a family. And when things got really bad, I consoled myself knowing that I also had Ben, a baby who had been a surprise only a year after Xander. I knew that Heavenly Father had given us Ben for a reason, and I knew what it was. It was to show us that even though things with Xander would be rough, we would be able to have the best of both worlds: the blessings that would come from raising Xander and the normalcy that would come from having Ben.

But then all of my understanding was gone. It made no sense to me that Heavenly Father's great plan for us would include two autistic children. That was not fair at all. And around the time that Ben was diagnosed, it seemed like nothing was going well for our family. My father-in-law had died suddenly at a young age, just after Xander had been diagnosed. And Xander had begun with his tantrum phase, just like any other preschooler. Well, except that Xander's tantrums lasted six hours, and we never knew what caused them. Sometimes, it could be because the lampshade was tilted funny or the stereo wasn't on the setting Xander wanted. It took us over a year to figure out how he wanted things. Xander could have a six-hour tantrum and several two-hour tantrums every day. We all walked on eggshells around him, afraid of setting him off.

Xander also couldn't tolerate having people over. He would scream the entire time anyone visited. As you can imagine, this greatly reduced our social lives.

And then it got to the point where we could no longer attend church. Xander was too disruptive, and we spent the whole time in the hallways. At first my husband and I alternated Sundays, but pretty soon we just rarely attended. I knew the decision was wrong, but at the time, I felt like we were living through a war, just doing what we could to survive. We rarely slept, and we spent most of our time listening to Xander scream. The only good thing in our lives was Ben. He was a delightful two-year old, and I remember worrying because he was too nice, too eager to share his toys. I worried that he was trying too hard to be the peacemaker in a family that was tearing apart.

So, shortly after Ben turned two, we felt like a family in crisis. We weren't attending church, we couldn't have home teachers or friends over and we were broke. It wasn't a great time in general, but I knew that it was only temporary. I still prayed fervently and read my scriptures, and I had absolute faith that Heavenly Father would bless us.

So it was no wonder that I felt so betrayed when things got even worse. Shortly after his second birthday, Ben changed. He became moody, easily frustrated and demanding. And then he stopped talking. Ben had always had a few language delays, and we easily attributed them to his frequent ear infections and the fact that his older brother didn't talk.

I never cried when they told me Xander was autistic. When they told me Ben was, I cried for two weeks straight. My mother listened to me as I wept over the phone, crying, "It's just not fair." She tried to help me see things positively, but I wasn't ready for it. The wound was so open and painful.

I can never explain my feelings for the first year we knew Ben was autistic. I remember feeling the most painful loneliness I've ever felt in my life. I still had some friends, and they were wonderful, but whenever I talked to them, I could only think about how their children were normal and mine weren't. It seemed like everyone else's life was working out perfectly, and mine was so hard.

I rarely went to church, but when I did, I just felt more bitter. There were people in our ward who had six, seven, even eight normal children. I just wanted one.

At this time, we had a new relief society president, a wonderful woman who never scolded me for being bitter. She seemed to understand that I just needed some time to feel sorry for myself. At the same time, she did what no one else had dared to: she asked me to provide service. And those times, when I helped her out, I felt the best I'd felt in a long time. This woman had so many problems of her own, and it helped me to know that there were some other people who were struggling.

Other than her, not too many people at church helped us out. It was hard not to be bitter, although looking back, there were few people who even knew what was going on, and fewer who knew what to do to help. I wasn't given callings for a while and the bishop was understanding about our not going to church. I know everyone had the best intentions and wanted to be helpful, but all of this made me feel like the people at church didn't care if we were part of the ward or not.

Things grew worse and worse. I developed horrible migraines that I had several times a week, and I began a horrible habit that even now, I am ashamed to even think about: I began screaming at the boys. It was hard not to resent them, though at the same time, I felt this tremendous love toward them. My self-esteem was the lowest it had ever been. All over the news and in magazines, there were these stories of incredible moms who had cured or made great progress in working with their autistic children. Mine were making remarkably slow progress, and I knew it was because I was doing everything wrong. All of my friends' children were talking and playing and getting potty-trained but not mine. I couldn't help but feel like a failure.

This is not to say that there weren't good moments during this time. Both boys went to developmental delay preschools, and I developed close relationships with their teachers and some of the other parents. I still had some friends, and my family was so supportive. My parents went way above and beyond to help out, often babysitting and giving us money.

The babysitting proved to be invaluable when things got even worse. All of a sudden, Xander got very attached to me. He'd always been somewhat attached, but it got to the point where if I left him with his father, he would cry the whole time. I couldn't make either Xander or

Joe put up with that, so I never left him. The only other person Xander would stay with was my mother, and if it weren't for that, I think I would have gone crazy. Still, the few things I attended, like enrichment night, had to stop, because I couldn't just leave Xander with Joe, and my mother babysat on days when I had to take Ben to the doctor and on Sundays if we wanted to go to church. I felt bad asking her to do more.

But the boys were making progress. Xander had gotten to the point where we could have people over and he no longer threw so many tantrums. We made the difficult decision to medicate him, and within days, he was a generally happy boy. He also started sleeping at least five hours a night. It's amazing how much better you can feel when you get some sleep.

Ben's progress was much more rapid. Xander hated having me work with him, his definition of what a mommy is was very clear, and mommies do not do work like teachers do. But Ben thought it was a treat to work with me. He started talking shortly before he turned three, and we discovered that sometime while he wasn't speaking, Ben learned his alphabet and how to read. He loved to draw and soon drew letters and then words. His language was delayed, but it was an incredible experience to hear him speak. You can't imagine how amazing it is to hear what is in your child's thoughts until that is taken away from you. Even when he was being obnoxious, I have delighted in knowing Ben's thoughts.

However, Ben's successes made me feel guilty for Xander's lack of it. I felt like I was failing him somehow, though looking back, I worked even harder at trying to communicate with Xander. We had, from the time Xander was diagnosed, looked into Applied Behavioral Analysis, an educational treatment for autism, but the costs of it were so beyond our means. We used other therapies, and tried some of the "cures" for autism, like a gluten-free and casein-free diet and vitamin supplements. It got to the point where I was spending $100 a month in vitamins alone. None of them worked, but we started Xander on horseback riding therapy, and we noticed immediate results. Xander was calmer and more willing to work with us.

After a while, we revisited the idea of ABA. It seemed a shame to deny him something just because of money. I prayed about the therapy and got a really good feeling. I tried to have faith that if this was right, Heavenly Father would provide the means.

My family became an invaluable resource to us. My grandmother paid for me and a friend of mine to get trained so we could work with

Xander, an aunt sent us money every month for the supplies and my mother put off retirement so Xander could have the therapy.

It was a struggle to get the program going, and we had a lot of setbacks, but we finally began the program when Xander was four and a half. This was late for starting ABA, but it worked out for us. I am not sure that Xander would have been ready to work any earlier.

It ended up that I couldn't work with Xander. He wouldn't have any parts of that, but we found another therapist. With her and my friend doing the program, we began to see some results. We never saw amazing breakthroughs, but we learned that Xander loves to do puzzles and that he enjoys matching things. We have gotten to know our son through this therapy, and that's been worth any price to me.

Ben still liked having me work with him, so I began doing language therapy with him. His progress was rapid and encouraging. Sometimes, one of Xander's therapists worked with Ben, and he was thrilled.

Then Xander went through an extremely hyper period. He would just jump up and down and scream. He slept for only two hours. Our household went in another period of unrest. We tried to live through it, but one day I discovered that Xander's heart rate was high. I brought him to the doctor, and his heart rate was more that double a normal rate. We tried many medications, but the only one that helped was Ritalin. Shortly after, Ben began exhibiting behavior problems. He was moody and intense, and often too keyed up. He would run away from school, and we couldn't take him anywhere because he couldn't behave well. He would knock things off of shelves at grocery stores, run away in the parking lots and scream loudly at restaurants. We tried putting him on medication, but nothing helped much.

During this time, I was literally at the end of my rope. I came to Heavenly Father in the most fervent prayer of my life. Things had to change, I knew. It was an incredibly spiritual experience as I learned to rely on Him. I began attending church again, and I often brought Ben. At three years old, he did well in sacrament meeting, considering he hadn't been in two years. Once I began attending, the Primary started to make arrangements for someone to take care of Xander during the Sunday school and Relief Society hours. Most of the time, this didn't work out. I tried to have faith.

Slowly, my faith began to increase and things got better. We brought Xander to an autism clinic in our state, and a doctor there told us that Xander was one of the happiest autistic kids he had met. Xander began attending kindergarten this fall in a self-contained autism classroom. He has made so much progress in the little time he's been there. He now understands basic commands, and eagerly follows them, which is more than could be said for a lot of "normal" five-year olds. He has a special helper at church who stays with him so his father and I can go to class. I recently bore my testimony about the love I have for Xander, and about how much it's taught me about Christ and His love for us. So many people came up and told me they had no idea I had two autistic children.

Ben attends a mainstreamed developmental delay preschool, and we have hopes that he will be able to go to regular kindergarten next year. He is extremely bright, though he still has delays. His obsessions drive us crazy, but behind them is a brilliant mind which eagerly attains knowledge. He can now make conversations, and while interacting with his peers is still hard for him, Ben is learning to make friends. He might always be someone who has trouble socially, but as his mother, I know I will always look at him and see how far he has come.

As I was struggling with my bitterness about our situation, I came across a scripture in John where Jesus is brought a blind man and asked, "Who has sinned, this man or his parents?" Jesus replies that neither has sinned but that the man is blind in order to show the works of God. I know that through my ordeals as the mother of two autistic boys, I have seen so many of those works.

There are times when it is hard, and when I get discouraged. My greatest struggle now has been the decision to have another child. As I pray, I haven't gotten an answer, and some of the old bitterness returned. Our finances have been depleted from the needs of the two children we have, and all doctors have recommended that we have no more natural children. We've looked into adoption, but we can't afford it. Recently, several friends have gotten pregnant. For the first ten people I heard about, I quietly offered congratulations, then hung up the phone and burst into tears. "Why?" I would challenge Heavenly Father. Sometime during this pregnancy streak, I began to feel uplifted by Him. I can't say that it's easy or that I understand it. But somehow, I retain the faith that even this will work out for the good of someone who loves Him, as we are promised in Romans.

The experiences I have had have sometimes flattened me, but some of them have been the most uplifting ones. I know that through my sons, Heavenly Father will work some great miracles. This was reiterated to me in Burger King the other day. I took the boys out, because they were driving me crazy, and I wanted to burn off some of their energy. They love to go to the play area in Burger King, and I usually try to go when it's not too busy. Some of the other kids can be cruel, and often the parents are even worse. This time, we were blessed to have the whole place to ourselves, and the boys were having a great time.

Then, a man came in with his two children. I was trying to ignore them, but the man brought his children up and introduced them to me. His daughter was Xander's age, and it was a little bit painful to see how much she talked. He asked me the names and ages of my children, and I told him. He told his children to say "hello" to my boys. I explained to the father that they were autistic and that Xander can't talk. The boy told Xander , "Hi," but Xander just replied with some loud sounds.

"Daddy," the boy said, "I told him 'hi,' but he's just making those weird noises."

"That's okay," said the father, "he hasn't learned to talk yet, so he makes those noises, but he knows you want to be his friend, and that's what's important."

I wish that more parents could teach their children such compassion, and I wish that more parents even had that compassion. I hope that wherever that man is, he knows what a special thing it is, that just one time, Xander was treated like a human being by a stranger.

I am so grateful that Heavenly Father has given us people like that man, people like my family, my friends and the dear Relief Society president who didn't wait for me to figure out what I needed. I am especially grateful for all of the special education teachers out there, who somehow decided to choose a profession where they would be completely selfless. Through all of these people, I have seen the works of God. I have learned the importance of charity and love, and after all, aren't those the greatest works He's created?

Chapter Four

Emma, age 4

Megan, age 13

by Lorena Jueschke

I don't remember my friend Deanna's exact words, but I do remember hearing the word, autism. How could that be? Her son Jonathan was so loving and sweet. Wasn't that the condition that made people cold and unattached? I thought it was really rare. Wasn't he supposed to be spinning or banging his head? He was just a little behind in talking and was unusually picky about food. You could say that about many children. And weren't there children that talked late who turned out to be geniuses?

I insisted that there was a less serious explanation. I did as I always did—I tried to alleviate fears by denying them. Hadn't I learned my lesson? This dear friend had always been right when she expressed concerns in the past, and I always tried to say it wasn't so. And, now, she was right about her son being autistic. Instead of being supportive from the beginning, I had to spend some time in denial. I should've acknowledged her fears and given them credence. My wishing them away with positive thinking wasn't going to make them invalid. The future would bring me a great lesson in this area.

Our fourth child came to us on a cool May, 1998, evening in the comfort of our own bed. The atmosphere was very calm and relaxed. We had our midwife, her assistant, and two doulas (mother's helpers) present. It hadn't even registered in my mind that our baby was almost here when I felt this soft, tiny body glide into my arms. The midwife immediately covered us both with a warmed blanket and I was the only one who could see those lovely eyes looking up at me. As David peaked in, I heard whispers asking if it was a boy or girl. That discovery was to be my right, and I was in no hurry. I was too mesmerized by that gaze to look away. I had a twinge of worry as I looked at that pixie-like face. I couldn't see any resemblance to our other three girls. Maybe that meant this baby was a boy? I finally lifted the blanket and announced that she was a girl! "Our little Emma! We have a quartet!" The room broke into "Ooooh's" and "Ahhhh's" and comments about the beautiful name. Suddenly, the midwife said, "This is a miracle baby!" Then she showed us the complete knot in Emma's umbilical cord. What a frightening thing that was to see. The midwife said, "This was why Emma picked today to be born." By the next day it could've been a truly dangerous thing. She mentioned how she was always amazed when the body seemed to know of impending disaster. This miracle turned out to be just the first unusual aspect of Emma. There would be many more to follow.

The three of us just snuggled there and our doulas served us a wonderful soup that my sister-in-law had brought. It was perfect. But, the midwife was watching Emma rather closely, and continued to suction her mucous frequently and provided oxygen. After an hour she began her follow-up, thorough examination, and she still wasn't happy with the amount of mucous Emma was struggling with. Emma was about to do something else that was unusual. The midwife explained that excess mucous is frequently a sign of infection, such as Strep B. This was something we shouldn't wait to see. She decided we needed to go to the hospital for testing. She believed they would admit Emma and observe her overnight.

But, before we left for the hospital, I wanted Emma to have a blessing; so we had my brother, who lived just a mile away, come over to help administer to her. The blessing David and my brother offered was truly inspired and the whole room was moved with the Spirit. Even the non-LDS midwife and doula believed that this blessing was given by God. On the way to the hospital one of the doulas, who had been a NICU nurse explained the wisdom of the midwife's recommendation and what would be happening when we arrived at the hospital. She was very reassuring. We were met at the door of the ER by the triage nurse who had prepared a bed for us. After she examined Emma, she announced that Emma's oxygen level was 98 and that you couldn't do much better than that. It was a big relief. The doctor seemed more curious about our mode of delivery than he was concerned for our baby's welfare. He did, however, call for the respiratory therapists from the NICU to make sure all was well. When they arrived and checked her, they believed that she had finally absorbed enough mucous and wasn't creating anymore, which meant that infection was unlikely. We were told that on rare occasions, babies take an excessive length of time to absorb the amniotic fluid. They didn't know why this happened, but there should be no ill effects. They declared that she was completely healthy, and they wished they got to see more like her. With that, the doctor dismissed us. We arrived home to find our house cleaned and our room dimly lit to make it cozy. Our assistants, then, tucked us into bed, and off we went to sleep.

I didn't set the alarm that night. After all, we had a new baby to wake us every few hours, right? But I awakened to see the sunlight peaking through the window. Oh no!!! My newborn baby had slept through the night and that meant she would be dehydrated. Would she be able to breastfeed if she was this weak? I tried not to go into a panic. But, prior experience had taught me that a baby that doesn't nurse enough in the first few days will become too weak to be motivated to eat. Our third daughter had dropped an alarming amount of weight as a newborn. It took six weeks to establish breastfeeding. We had to seek the assistance of a lactation consultant. I liked to call her, "Linda, the Lactation Lady". We became experts on breastpumps.

So, now you know the wacky concerns going through my mind as I looked at Emma. When she was less than a day old, I knew already that we'd have an uphill battle with breastfeeding. I once had a doctor tell me that many babies would rather sleep than eat. I guess Emma was one of those. I was never going to watch another baby lose so much weight again, though. I called Linda immediately and told her my concerns. I began pumping that day. Emma never needed formula, but it was nearly impossible for her to gain weight by nursing. She just ate too slowly. After two months of trying everything we'd tried with Marissa, I felt Emma had decided to be bottlefed. I was still nursing at night because the doctor thought she was getting enough during the day that she'd be okay overnight with fewer calories. So, we had a plan and it was working. Little did we know, Emma was going to do something that our very experienced lactation consultant had never seen happen. At six months, Emma refused to take the bottle and couldn't be consoled except by nursing. Would she get enough milk to be healthy, though? I contacted the doctor and Linda again to ask for advice. After several weeks of frequent weight checks and recording solid food intake in detail, it was determined that she was perfectly fine with breastfeeding. This was an amazing development. It didn't occur to me that this could be a sign of something amiss.

We noticed that Emma couldn't be held by anyone except David or me. She didn't like her sisters to touch her. I can remember the most common chastisement I made against our other girls was to "Leave Emma alone!" It seemed I had to say this a hundred times a day. My mother-in-law, who our children refer to as Mimi, would comment that Emma was so temperamental. That was true. I can remember feeling like I had to do back-flips to encourage a smile out of her. But, for her to reject her grandmothers was painful for them to experience and painful for me to witness. I remember a time when my father-in-law, who the children call Poppi, was holding her. He has a silly way about him with all his funny faces, and Emma finally cracked a momentary smile. Mimi was so jealous. She said to Poppi, "How must you rank?" But, of course, this stoic tendency in Emma was just her personality, I would reason.

When Emma was nine months old, events took a bad turn. She virtually stopped eating, and all the strides she'd made in smiling ceased. I knew she must be sick, but there were no clear signs of illness. It wasn't my first thought to run to the doctor. After all, she probably just had a cold, and doctors can't be much help with a cold. But, when her weight started to drop and she developed a deep cough, we had to see what was happening. We were in the process of selecting a new pediatrician. We'd never tried out a new doctor with a sick child before, but that couldn't stop us this time. We learned that maybe that's the best way to try out a new doctor. He was great! Emma had bronchitis, and the doctor determined that she had asthma. I was a little surprised. Unfortunately, Emma turned out to be allergic to penicillin. She broke out in hives from head to toe. Thankfully, she responded well to the sulfa drugs.

I began to associate all her moody behavior with asthma. If she was crying in a store, she must be wheezing. If she wasn't sleeping at night, she must need her medicine. When she was throwing a fit during our entire trip to Washington for David's family reunion, it must've been because of allergies to all those trees. I relied on that diagnosis to explain everything. But, then, David's cousin had a son with asthma. He was about the same age as Emma. The whole time we were there, he had one episode of hives after another. He was so allergic to everything that he made Emma's allergies seem non-existent. At the same time, this little boy was the happiest little guy you can imagine. Why was that? Was I just kidding myself that Emma's fussiness was all because of her asthma?

Emma didn't walk until she was 17 months old. At the time, I thought it was because I held her so much (which, of course, was because she was so touchy). Or, maybe, it was because the floor wasn't a safe place for a baby to be adventurous due to the three, older girls leaving their toys around. Maybe it was because I didn't trust her to be on the floor where she could put every little scrap or object into her mouth.

The doctor felt that she was still within the normal range and comforted my concerns. But, at the same time, I began to over-estimate Emma's milestones. The doctor asked if she was saying a few words. Of course, she'd said some words. I just didn't point out that she only used them once, and then we never heard them again. He asked if she was jumping and running. Well, sure, but I didn't mention that she leaned to the side when she ran and that she only jumped if you were bouncing her. Did she wave? "Sure," I'd say. But, I should've mentioned that this would happen after the people were already a block away. I don't know why I was so protective of her deviations from the norm. Maybe it was because I was afraid that her problems would all be blamed on me? Or maybe they'd say it was because she was born at home? (I'd gotten a lot of comments about that choice.) Maybe it was because I'd damaged her psyche with all my efforts to breastfeed? Or was it that she was our fourth child and I was too tired or incompetent to have so many children? Was it because I worked as a computer programmer from home? Did we miss some pivotal developmental stage when her older sister got sick with Graves' Disease (hyperthyroidism), and we were a bit preoccupied for a while getting her stabilized? There were so many possibilities, and they all pointed to a failure in me. I'd like to think that I wasn't so selfish as to avoid addressing Emma's problems just because I didn't want to look bad; but I believe this inward fear was at the core of why I chose, instead, to believe that Emma was just developing at her own pace, within the normal sphere.

In the meantime, Emma had developed some cute idiosyncrasies that we found enjoyable and never thought to be disturbing. David is a funeral director/mortician. He had long made a practice of removing his work shoes in the garage before entering the house because he didn't want to bring chemicals or germs in with him. Emma found this to be a problem. She couldn't tolerate his wearing his socks without his shoes. David didn't like walking around the house with his shoes or slippers on, but he did like to wear his socks. She'd bring him shoes and start putting them on his feet no matter how hard he resisted. When this became too much of a problem, David stopped leaving his shoes outside. Then, she started following him to the bedroom and wouldn't let him take his shoes off at all. What a genius she was! Of course, it doesn't make sense to wear socks without shoes!

She also took great pains in making sure that my shirt wasn't bunched up in the back. She'd come up to me countless times in a day and realign my blouse. I thought it was nice that she was developing a sense of style.

She didn't like sand. She wouldn't step on it. She seemed to think it was like water and that she was going to sink into it. Even if I was carrying her while walking across sand, she was afraid. As annoying as this fear was, it also seemed very astute to me. The fact that she hated the swing just meant that I wasn't going to have to stand there and push her in it for hours (as I recalled doing with the other girls).

Then there were eating issues. While she wasn't picky about what she ate, she was picky about how she ate it. From the time she had her first solid food at six-months-old, she insisted on touching her food. I was never able to spoon food into her mouth. This habit could drive you nuts if you were a stickler for a clean floor! Imagine the mess from things like rice cereal. I just chalked this up to her scientific exploration of the world around her. None of these things added up to something serious in my mind.

I suppose Emma had become notorious in the ward for her high-pitched scream. During Stake Conference she screamed so loud I had to leave the stand (I was the Stake choir accompanist) to take her out of the building and walk down the block in order not to disturb the meeting. David was seated in the middle with the choir and couldn't get to her quickly enough. That turned out to be a zinger, since I didn't return in time to accompany the primary choir. In the future, we found she did better if we sat in the front and she couldn't see all the people. These kinds of incidences were probably why the first day of nursery amazed everyone. She just walked right in there and didn't even notice me leaving. When I arrived in Sunday School without her, everyone that saw me alone said they were surprised that she went into the nursery so well. I admitted to them that I was just as surprised. But, it did make me wonder how others were perceiving her.

One Sunday, the nursery leader's husband was helping her. He's a third-grade teacher. He asked me if I'd noticed that Emma didn't answer to her name. It hadn't really occurred to me that I didn't call her name and expect her to come. I usually just went to her. He suggested that she may be deaf or hard-of-hearing. I hadn't thought of that—especially since she seemed to wake up if I dropped a rag! It was true, however, that the vacuum didn't even startle her. Unlike our other girls, Emma would walk right up to the vacuum. So, maybe deafness was as reasonable an explanation for her behavior as my asthma theory.

We contacted the doctor for a referral for a hearing test. He thought that would be a good idea since she still wasn't talking. But, he was convinced that she was just reacting to having three, older sisters who were probably doing all the talking for her. That sounded reasonable. I can remember talking for my younger brother. After the hearing evaluation we were told that it wasn't conclusive and we should get a BAER test. This would be done by placing probes on her head and measuring her brain wave reaction to sounds while under general anesthetic. We went to Children's Hospital in Los Angeles for the test. It was kind of eerie walking into this huge hospital. I knew this was where my older brother had died six weeks after I was born. He was almost 3 years old and died of leukemia. For some reason, this knowledge made me feel sad just walking in the door. As we were signing in, the doctor suggested that before we do the BAER test, they should try to do a standard hearing test. I reminded them that the routine test had already been done, but the doctor responded that they have ways of making it more effective. Maybe we'd get lucky and not have to conduct the BAER test.

Well, after the test the doctor came in and told us that not only was Emma's hearing fine, but it appeared to be far superior to mine! I guess they could tell which sounds I didn't hear. We were able to skip the BAER test. As we walked into the reception area I saw a huge poster about autism. I tried to ignore it. But, now that we knew Emma had perfect hearing, what could be the problem? We asked the doctor what we should do next. She counseled us to have a speech evaluation as soon as possible.

By this time Emma was over two years old. The insurance company suggested that we go to our local hospital for the speech evaluation. The therapist was a sweet, young woman. She met with us in the physical therapy department of the hospital and took us into a small office that seemed more like a big closet. She had some toys under her desk and there wasn't much room on the floor, but that was clearly the best place to conduct the test. When she finished, she announced that Emma's expressive language abilities were only in about the six-month age range. I was stunned. How could this be? Six-month-olds don't say words, but Emma said words occasionally. She explained that she could only grade up a level if most of the areas in a level had been reached. Emma had some skills in higher levels, but this was her determination overall. I was scared to death. What did this mean? How do we fix it? She suggested that she might not be the best therapist for Emma since she didn't have the best facilities to work with children. But, she could work with her until we arranged for her to go to a place called Baby Steps. There she would be involved in early intervention. She also suggested that we contact the Regional Center. Well, this name was entirely too vague—the regional center of what? What on earth is a Regional Center? Her explanation left me even more confused. Then I remembered Deanna dealing with the Regional Center with some level of frustration. It was at this moment I realized that I hadn't paid nearly enough attention when she was talking about her struggles to get help for her son. I remember feeling bad that she had to run all over town with paperwork that never seemed to end. But, I didn't understand much of it. It turns out that the Regional Center is a pretty simple concept. In California, it's the entity that helps the developmentally disabled. There are other states that use this model, also. They don't just help those that have a diagnosis. They help children that are showing signs they may be at risk of some of these problems. Through early intervention, the child might keep from falling behind.

The Regional Center case worker came to our home for Emma's evaluation. If Emma qualified, they would pay for her to receive therapies through Baby Steps. I remember asking her if she thought Emma was autistic. She said that professionals would be brought in to make those sorts of assessments. I explained that Emma couldn't be autistic because one of my best friends had an autistic child and that was just too many statistically in a group to be logical. She gave me the strangest look. But, I honestly thought my idea made a lot of sense. You have to remember though, I'm a computer programmer. That's just how my mind works. At the time I viewed autism as a mysterious and rare condition. The chances of two children like this in a group of friends seemed impossible. That was my protection. Our whole world was about to change.

Baby Steps' assessments found that Emma required speech therapy, occupational therapy, and mommy-me type classes. This schedule sent my head spinning. Many of the moms I talked to were overwhelmed by this schedule, but I felt particularly drained by it. I was the Relief Society secretary at the time. This calling wasn't horribly time-consuming, but everything about the new schedule seemed to be too much for me. I was also the choir accompanist, but I was having trouble dragging myself out of bed on Sunday mornings in time. Working from home required that I have things running pretty smoothly at home. But I felt like my life was spinning out of control.

My dad was a high school choir teacher. I'd promised to accompany for his first two classes Monday - Thursday that last year before his retirement. There was the preschool schedule for our 4-year-old and the homework for our other two girls. It didn't seem like a lot on paper, but it felt like an amusement park ride. The worst part of it all was that Emma didn't seem to be learning anything with all these therapies. The best I could report was that she'd learned not to scream through everything, but I never lost hope. For some reason, I just assumed that things were going to improve immensely.

Emma was two months away from turning three, when the Regional Center conducted their evaluations. We started out with a medical evaluation. The doctor was very interested in Emma's facial features. It was her pixie-like face that I think had him so intrigued. He wanted us to see a geneticist at UCLA to rule out conditions such as Fragile X. In my heart I knew the problem wasn't any of these genetic defects, but I did want to research all the possibilities; and we had a very interesting meeting with the UCLA geneticist. In the end, though, it seemed like we were there more for the doctors' research than for Emma's benefit. They couldn't tell us anything except that the problem wasn't a known genetic condition.

Next was the psychological evaluation. This doctor went through a "mile" of questions for David and me. At the same time she seemed to be watching Emma's every move. At one point David described how Emma needed to "caress" her food, especially soft foods like ice cream. The doctor's eyes got really big, and this information seemed significant. Then she asked us if Emma needed to line things up. We'd never noticed her doing that. Just then the doctor pointed out that Emma was lining up the ends of her papers and had been doing that for the last five minutes. Her observations were all very interesting, but I really didn't know what to think of all that.

One day at our Baby Steps class the teacher mentioned the Autism Society of America's (ASA) conference that would be held that weekend in Pasadena. She asked if all of us moms would be attending. Several of us hadn't heard anything about it. She gave us each copies of the information and told us to call our Regional Center case workers to have them arrange it. I asked if they would do this even if our child didn't have a diagnosis of autism. The teacher looked at me pretty seriously and said that they would set it up for me. I sensed that she knew something I hadn't been told. I called my case worker to make the request. She said she'd requisition it right away. I then double-checked with her that it would be alright even without the diagnosis. It was then that she got really quiet and told me that the report was being mailed to me, but the finding was that it was autism. I couldn't believe I was hearing this news over the phone this way. They didn't even call me. I was calling them. I'm sure I already knew it was autism. I just imagined we'd hear the news in a different way. Tears suddenly welled up.

My logical mind began trying to figure out why I would be crying over news I already knew. I don't know why I didn't feel that crying was a reasonable thing to do, but I had a really hard time just letting myself do it. I immediately called David to tell him. Everything after that felt like a blur. I recalled a moment years before. As a pianist, I would sometimes just go through the hymn book or the primary song book and play things I hadn't heard. I came upon a primary song that brought me to uncontrollable tears. The words, "I'll walk with you. I'll talk with you. That's how I'll show my love for you.," seemed to burn into my soul. I don't know why this song affected me so much on that day. I had no idea they would someday mean everything to me... Remembering this moment, I sought out that song and played it over and over.

Going to the conference was overwhelming, to say the least. I hadn't had time to adjust to this diagnosis yet, and here I was hearing in-depth lectures on the subject. I was like a sponge and absorbed so much that I just oozed out information to David when I got home. I attended with my friend, Deanna. Her son had been diagnosed four years earlier. Since it appeared that he was on the high-functioning end of the spectrum, she chose to attend classes for a condition called, "Asperger's Syndrome." I attended classes geared more toward classic autism. Afterward, we went out to dinner and compared notes. The first thing Deanna told me about her classes was that they had described my oldest daughter, Megan, to a tee.

Megan was born in September, 1989. She was the most beautiful baby I'd ever seen. Her head was absolutely perfect, in part because she was born by Cesarean section. She had piercing blue eyes and an easy-going temperament. She had really given us a scare though. When I was five months pregnant, she stopped moving. Examination found that Megan's heart rate wasn't very consistent, which the doctor assured me was probably a sign of her reacting to the monitor. He gave me a fetoscope for home to use anytime I hadn't felt her move for a while. He also sent us directly to the perinatologist's office for examination. They didn't know exactly what the problem was, but they suspected that Megan might have spina-bifida. This suggestion was terribly frightening to us. My only consolation was that the AFP blood test they administered early in pregnancy didn't show risk for this condition. They wanted to do an amniocentisis to know for sure. David and I prayed about it over the weekend. I received a blessing, and we prepared for this somewhat risky procedure. When we arrived at the doctor's office he informed us that the perinatologists were not recommending the test due to the amount of amniotic fluid and that they really thought spina-bifida was unlikely. I went in, during my lunch hour from work, twice a week for ultrasounds and non-stress tests for the rest of the pregnancy. Toward the end Megan found the transverse position (lying across my body) to be the most comfortable. I could feel her head wedged into my rib cage. After her surgical delivery the doctor held my hand and said, "She's just perfect." I knew she would be all along—even though the doctors were scaring me to death.

Megan was the easiest baby imaginable. She seemed to be born on a perfect schedule. I attributed that to the hospital schedule though, since we were there for five days. She didn't care if she was bottle-fed or breast-fed, and she started getting bottles the first day. I was convinced that all the hoopla about nipple confusion was just a bunch of hooey because of that. Anyone could hold her. She just loved the attention. I attributed that to the fact that I worked full time, so she was with other people a lot. It sure made her a popular baby in the ward. She could sit through entire concerts without making any kind of fuss. I always thought it was funny when people would go on and on about her attention span and how well-behaved she was at these adult functions.

I should've been alarmed when she started crawling on her back, like a crab, instead of on her hands and knees, but it didn't dawn on me that this action could be a neurological problem. I simply thought it was just her individuality. When she was under two she could sit through an entire opera. All of her grandparents are opera "nuts." They each told us of occasions when she would sit for three hours, just mesmerized by the music. We were sure she was musically gifted. I recorded in her baby book that she could sing long before she could talk. One Sunday she gave our ward a jolt when she burst out in song at the chorus of "I Stand All Amazed." She couldn't really even talk yet; and there she was belting out, "Oh, it is wonderful that He should care for me enough to die for

58

me. Oh, it is wonderful, wonderful to me." Megan didn't really say single words. She just started right out speaking in full sentences when she was about two years old. She had an interesting way of wording things, too. For instance, she would call pantyhose, "panty toes." She'd also say, "I hurt I-self." And the one that lingers still today is, "I have full hands." Rather than constantly correcting her, I would leave these phrases alone because I didn't want to discourage her from talking by nit-picking her speech.

Then she started preschool. My sister-in-law, Dawn, had a home-based preschool that Megan attended. Now, you need to know that my nieces and nephew are unusually bright. When Dawn said that Megan seemed a little bit spacey and immature, I assumed she was comparing my typical child to her gifted ones; and, of course, there would be no comparison. It didn't really occur to me that she may have been comparing Megan to the other, typical preschoolers she worked with. Her unusual behavior could be rationalized away with the argument that Megan was a particularly artistic child and that would make her more sensitive.

Her first-grade teacher was convinced Megan had ADHD; and half-way had us convinced, too. But that diagnosis just didn't seem to fit. Our pediatrician suggested that maybe there was just a personality conflict between Megan and the teacher. She advised us to see how she related to the next teacher. At the same time, her primary teacher noted that Megan wrote everything mirror-image backwards. We had noticed this and thought maybe it was a product of her being left-handed. This was yet another example of my making senseless things make sense. Now we could see that her behavior was truly puzzling. She didn't seem to have dyslexia, but it had to be something like that. You could hold almost everything she wrote up to a mirror and read it. We were told that it should cease by the time she entered third grade; and if not, then they would address it more aggressively. Now, I look back on that episode and think we were far too complacent about it. It was a major sign that something was wrong.

Second grade brought a nice change. This teacher seemed to understand Megan and saw her odd behaviors as artistic. That alleviated our fears of ADHD, and we never considered it again as a possibility. However, there was no denying that Megan performed very poorly on the standardized tests. I figured that she just wasn't academically gifted. She was very musical and artistic, and it made sense to me that you can't have everything. As long as she was doing her best with her school work, I didn't worry. She was a very hard worker.

The third grade teacher encouraged a sweet girl in her class to spend time with Megan. I appreciated this because Megan was so shy. We would walk down the hall at school, and every child we'd pass would say, "Hi, Megan!" But she wouldn't even look their way. This teacher believed that Megan was very unusual, but she never indicated exactly how. Megan's backward writing began to disappear, so all concerns about it also disappeared. This teacher was very helpful to Megan, so Megan had a good year. This didn't change the fact, however, that she continued to perform terribly on the standardized tests. All the while, she was receiving pretty good grades. I could never make sense of this. Either they were grading purely on effort, and our girl was falling behind; or she was just a really poor test taker. When I'd ask about this at school, I was always told it was fine.

Sixth grade brought a turning point. This was the beginning of middle school and that meant a completely different kind of environment. These children were now into "style" like never before. Megan detested the concept of style. She just liked to be comfortable. She had no tolerance for people who broke rules, and she was always in trouble for "tattling." She also had great difficulty playing games. This made her the object of constant teasing.

The teacher felt that Megan would do fine if she could just keep from crying. We knew it was a good day if Megan came home and said, "I didn't cry at all today." But, this was also the year we started Emma with Baby Steps. I couldn't focus a lot of attention on Megan's social difficulties beyond that. It was something she would just have to work out. I remembered junior high as a very difficult time socially; but I also remember that I learned a lot about social behavior during that time. I chalked it all up to growing pains.

As spring came around, Megan began showing signs of severe depression. She was sad all the time and was dwelling on death. Now, I could rationalize that the daughter of a mortician wasn't going to shy away from the subject of death, but in truth, this dark mood was more than just being comfortable with the subject. She was wondering why she had to continue to live. Then we got Emma's diagnosis and I went to the conference. I began to wonder if all of Megan's problems really could be stemming from an autistic tendency.

I called for a student study meeting with the school. All of her teachers, the vice-principal, Megan, and I were present. We went around the table and each teacher laid out Megan's strengths and weaknesses. The choir teacher was the most positive about Megan. You could tell that she really loved Megan. I also knew that this class was the only good thing happening for Megan at school. The PE teacher was less optimistic. He found that Megan was somewhat uncoordinated and that she had trouble with the rules of the games. She also had a temper when she didn't play well, but he hadn't seen any incidents of ridicule in class and his perception was that the kids were very patient with her.

Megan disagreed. However, she didn't make a big issue of it at the meeting, nor did she offer any examples of the problems she was having there. Then it came around to her academic teacher. She, essentially, said that Megan was doing well in all her subjects, but had a tendency to forget to turn in assignments. The teacher would find the assignments in Megan's desk, completed. It was puzzling to the teacher, since she claimed she was always reminding the class to turn in their work. This was frustrating to me because it was completely out of my control. Unlike homework, which I could monitor, during school time Megan was on her own. The thought came across that Megan still needed a lot of hand-holding. I brought this up, and it was met with astonishment. I could see they just figured me for an over-protective parent. The vice-principal said that Megan was too old for such hand-holding. It was time for her to develop more independence. While I agreed with this idea basically, it seemed impossible to accomplish. Just saying it was so wasn't going to make it so. But the recommendation decided upon at that time was that Megan should keep a calendar and work on her organizational skills.

I was very frustrated because I wanted a psychological evaluation to find out what was really happening. I walked out with the vice-principal and asked her if she thought it was possible that Megan had ADHD or maybe some form of autism since her sister was autistic. The vice-principal told me that clearly Megan had control over her attention span or she wouldn't be able to focus so clearly on the things she was interested in. That seemed to rule out ADHD; and as far as autism, that seemed to be a total stretch to her. Essentially, the vice-principal felt I was overreacting. Megan went off-track a few days later because she went to a year-round school. During the break I talked to her pediatrician about her depression; and he felt that if anything, I wasn't reacting enough. He advised me to get help for her as soon as possible.

I contacted the insurance company to find out what our options were for a psychiatrist. None of them felt right to me. We decided to pray about it, but no answer came (which we interpreted to mean that we shouldn't consider the psychiatrist at this time). Instead, we noticed that being away from school made Megan much happier. We started to see her smiling again. She stopped talking about death so much. I began researching home-schooling. There were lots of ways we could do it. We could buy books and fill out paperwork with the state and just do what we wanted. That seemed overwhelming to me both financially and practically. The next option was to go through the school district. The good thing would be that we'd have lots of help. The bad thing was that they'd tell us what to learn and when to have it done. That seemed to defeat part of my purpose, since the whole idea was to tailor this more to Megan's needs. So, we chose to go with a charter school that oversees homeschoolers. They were chartered through a public school district so we would have all the transcript documentation. But, they allowed the parents freedom to make all the curriculum decisions and go at their own pace. We also were assigned an educational specialist (ES) who monitored our progress, handled all the district paperwork, and helped us find resources. The charter school also offered group instruction for certain subjects. Within a few weeks of homeschooling Megan asked if she could always be taught at home. She loved it. I enrolled her in a PE class, sign language, drama, and choir. All of these wonderful, homeschooled children were very kind to her; and she got the social time she needed so that she would not completely lose touch with people.

Our ES conducted some placement testing to determine a starting point. This testing showed that she really was very far behind in many areas. At the same time she had an advanced vocabulary, even though she didn't seem to have the pragmatics of speech going for her. This puzzled the person giving the test; and it proved to me that, even though we were addressing the symptoms pretty well, we still needed to find the source of the problems.

Megan had just turned twelve a few days before her evaluation with Regional Center. We knew the drill. We'd been through it all before. But this time I was sure they would think I was nuts for bringing her there. The physical exam only showed that she was, indeed, healthy. He asked her some math questions for her to solve in her head. She had extreme difficulty with this and answered incorrectly each time. I figured she was pretty typical at this since I've always been bad at figuring math in my head even though I'm kind of a math whiz. I imagined that, when we left, he was laughing about my bringing this perfectly healthy girl in to see him. Then it was time for the psychological evaluation. Normally with a child Megan's age they like the parents to wait outside, since their presence can alter the child's answers. But I knew Megan would do better just knowing I was there. Besides, I really was curious as to how this was conducted. I promised to sit behind Megan out of her view and not do anything to distract her if I stayed. The doctor gave me a questionnaire to fill out at the same time. As I listened to the evaluation I kept thinking that Megan was completely normal and I must look like some kind of hypochondriac for bringing her in for this exam. I had no idea what some of the tests were looking for, but Megan seemed to me to be doing very well. When it was all over, the doctor asked Megan to go to the waiting room so she could talk to me. I figured that she wanted to talk to me right away because there wasn't a problem and she didn't want me to have to wait to know that. After all, we didn't get Emma's diagnosis for two months, and I had to call in to find that out. She closed the door and blurted out that Megan was definitely on the autism spectrum. She would have to evaluate the test results, but she thought it would come back in the Aspergers' Syndrome range. I was astounded! To top it all off she stated that Megan's IQ was in the low-normal range. I felt an immediate pain in my heart. Did this mean that my genius daughter was actually slow? She would never make the best grades? She probably wouldn't get that college scholarship that I was hoping for?

When all my friends were talking about their gifted children there was a reason I felt like crawling under a rock. The doctor pointed out that Megan was a very hard worker and that it was hard work for her every day as she tried to comprehend the things she heard, read, or saw. She had a great imagination, however; and she needed to focus her attention on her gifts, which were music and drama. The doctor could see the level of disappointment I was experiencing. She asked what was making this report the hardest? I told her it was all about me. It was because I was an over-achiever from a young age. Since I had been five years old I had been in the gifted program at school. Good grades were always just a matter of effort for me. I couldn't understand working so hard and still only getting a "C." That's when the doctor pointed out to me that a "C" is average, not a disaster. Being average is perfectly acceptable, and Megan was certainly capable of this. The doctor told me to put it in perspective.

Megan was not mentally retarded, and she had great potential (which can't always be said when autism is the diagnosis).

At that moment I realized how misplaced all my feelings about motherhood were. It has nothing to do with producing the most capable people. It's all about helping a child reach his own individual potential. You can't measure the success of the parent on the level of achievement of the child. This was the "yuppie" mentality that we started our family in. The truth was that our success was going to be measured on the level of happiness our children experienced and that would come from helping them find their gifts.

Megan was too old not to tell her the diagnosis. She knew we were seeing all these people for a reason. She also knew this was where we'd taken Emma. The doctor told us to tell Megan right away. David and I didn't know what to do. We prayed about it that evening and took Megan aside immediately. She seemed so relieved to know that the thing that had made her feel so different all her life was something that other people dealt with, too. I didn't want this "label" to become her excuse, but at the same time I wanted her to use this label to help us help her. We had horrible guilt about the expectations we'd had.. At the same time, these same expectations had helped her live a relatively typical life up to this point. But now, we'd know why she struggled so much and our goal from here on out would be to take this into consideration during those frustrating moments.

The young women in our ward have proven to be exceptional in many respects. They have always been kind and patient with Megan. Rather than teasing her when she gets overwhelmed they lovingly put their arms around her and pave the way for her to reach the goal. This was really evident at girls' camp. The plan was to go rappelling. Now, it makes a lot of sense that this activity would scare her. It's pretty scary to trust a rope while stepping off a high rock. But I also knew that this would be a wonderful challenge for Megan to overcome. At the same time, it wasn't worth "freaking her out" about. So, I told the leaders to encourage Megan a little bit on this, but let it go if she put up much of a fuss. I think the camp director was so inspired that day. She tricked Megan to the top of the rock by telling her that she just wanted to take her picture at the top, since she wasn't going to be able to get her coming down. When they got to the top Megan turned to her and said, "Okay. Take the picture." It was then that the camp director realized that she didn't bring the camera with her. Well, since they were up there, maybe Megan should just go ahead and rappel down. Megan took one look over the side and gave an emphatic, "No!" That was enough. They walked back down.

The other girls told Megan that it was really fun, but they could see why she was afraid. Megan turned out to be the only one that didn't rappel. During the testimony meeting Megan announced that next year she would do it! Everyone in the group cheered her. Now, this doesn't sound like typical testimony meeting behavior to me, but this meant something at this moment. It was support from her peers, and I appreciate these girls no end for it.

Megan's next challenge came during a Sunday School lesson she received about gaining your own testimony. By the time we saw Megan after church she was in full-blown tears. She was so upset, she couldn't talk until we got home. I took her into the bedroom and asked her to describe what was going on. She then divulged to me that she was not in the right place. She didn't know if she had a testimony. These heart-felt concerns should be common among children her age. For Megan it was intolerable. I very much respected her desire to gain a testimony. But, I was concerned that a testimony would be hard for her to come by with her literal thinking. For instance, the scriptures had always puzzled her. She was always trying to figure out how these stories were literally going to play out in her life.

So, we discussed how a testimony is gained by study and prayer. I also told her that until she had her own, it was perfectly fine for her to rely on her father's and mine. This seemed to ease her concerns for the day, but the next morning she began fretting about it all over again. We pulled out the scriptures, and I directed her to all the scriptures that talk about personal revelation and gaining a testimony. I then told her that it was okay if a testimony didn't happen all at once. I told her about how I gained my testimony. I was about thirteen. I read the Book of Mormon and, when I got to the end, I fasted for a day and ended my fast with a series of prayers. I told her of the deep warmth I felt as I prayed. I prayed about Joseph Smith and felt even more warmth as I seemed to see in my own mind the things that transpired. Then I prayed about Christ's atonement for our sins and it was at that time I felt the strongest warmth yet. It's a feeling I've never been able to shake or deny, and it has sustained my testimony all these years.

So, she sought to follow the same path. Megan felt a lot of distress. Reading the Book of Mormon (or any scripture) causes her great anxiety. David and I took turns answering her questions as she read. One day she just decided out of the blue to fast. I saw her head to her room where she stayed for quite a while. When she emerged, she was very upset. It hadn't happened! She didn't have the burning in her bosom. She said, "It must not be true!"

I didn't know what to say. Each person is entitled to his own revelation. I took her back in her room, and I told her we'd pray together. This time I wanted her to ask specific questions, the way I'd done as a girl. When she was done she turned to me with tears in her eyes, and she told me that she did feel it. She just didn't realize that's what I was talking about when I described a burning in the bosom. She thought it would be more like fire.

Well, this was a definite "Aspie" moment, but, she was so relieved to "find" her testimony. At the next Fast and Testimony meeting she bore her testimony in a simple and poignant way. When she stood up, David and I looked at each other with the kind of panic you feel when your young child might divulge some stupid thing you've done. We thought of all the embarrassing things she could say or do. Instead, she seemed to be guided and inspired with each word she uttered. Her whole countenance seemed transformed. I doubt many in that room understood the monumental thing that occurred in that meeting. For those of us who knew of Megan's struggles, this was a most spiritual manifestation.

Meanwhile, our case worker, Lori, recommended respite services to give us a little break from Emma. I couldn't imagine that getting a break from her would be anything good for me. She was so sensitive that leaving her with anyone was horribly stressful. Lori told me that we could use an agency or we could select our own respite worker as long as the person was 18 or older. I hung up the phone with her and began praying to know who should take care of our little girl.

A few moments later the phone rang. A young woman from our ward asked me to accompany her for a solo she was going to sing to earn her "Young Women in Excellence" award. I'd seen Lila exemplify many lovely traits in the past. Her wanting to sing a solo endeared her even more to me. She was one of my father's students in the high school choir, and she was a straight "A" student.

Suddenly I thought that she might be the exact type of girl to take on the challenge. I asked her when she'd be turning 18. She answered that she'd turned 18 the prior week! Then I asked her what she'd be studying in college and where she was planning to attend. (There was no point in getting her started with us if she was going to leave in a few months.) She said that she planned to attend the local community college for at least a year before transferring to an out-of-state university and that she'd be pursuing deaf studies. She wanted to work with deaf children..

Well, this was just too coincidental. I still needed to see how she'd feel about the job. I explained everything about it to her and asked her if she'd be interested. She was so happy to comply, and we set up a schedule. Emma loved Lila immediately. Lila became an integral part of our family. (Too bad her parents wouldn't let us steal her away as our own daughter. I guess they loved her, too! Oh well. This didn't stop us from loving her like she was our own.)

Upon turning 3, Emma needed to start special education pre-school. Regional Center set up the meetings with the school. I was very confused about how this would help her. I was convinced that she needed one-on-one therapy. I'd read about something called ABA or Applied Behavioral Analysis. Some people I talked to discounted the value of this therapy, saying it was like dog training, but it made so much sense to me that Emma needed something that typical children don't need. If it came in the form of "dog-training," I didn't care.

There were rumors that the Regional Center was paying for DTT (Discrete Trial Training), which is the portion of ABA that we needed, but, they were only doing it with children younger than three. That was because after age three, the school district was supposed to be responsible. DTT consists of breaking down tasks into parts and using drills to teach them. So, coming into the first meeting with the school, I was ready with my request for them to fund DTT. They looked at me like I was speaking French! The psychologist had worked at UCLA with Dr. Lovaas, the father of ABA, and she insisted that ABA wasn't what Emma needed. ABA only worked in therapy at a table with the therapist and wasn't very successfully generalized. I insisted that ABA was something I wanted to try and see if Emma responded positively to it. The psychologist then took me aside and told me that if I submitted a clear letter about the results I hoped to see from DTT and made them all behavioral then the Regional Center would have to fund it. This turned out to be a brilliant ploy by the school district. At that point, the issues we had were behavioral, so I had no problem using this method as our starting point. I knew, however, that there would eventually be a fight when Emma's issues became academic.

I submitted my letter of request to the Regional Center. Our wonderful case worker was so impressed that we should get this service that she kept us as her case even though she was supposed to move us on when Emma turned three. She wanted to see us through the process of getting DTT. Emma was three years and four months old when we met with our therapists, Celena and Yesenia, and their supervisor. These young women were all college students who had an interest in childhood development and had been trained by a psychologist in DTT.

Eventually we added Erika to the mix. I was amazed at how suddenly this service rolled into our life. They were in our home 15 hours a week. Emma was in school three hours a day. You'd think that this would've freed up hours for me, but it didn't feel that way at all. Having all these people in our home made me very aware of how time was divided. Emma learned at an astonishing rate. In only a few weeks they taught her to "sit down." This feat was a major accomplishment, since at that point she was unable to follow any instruction without physical prompting. We had our proof that DTT was going to be highly effective with her. The girls working with her used only positive reinforcement, and we learned quickly that she didn't need anything more than enthusiastic praise. All the negative things I'd been told about DTT using punishments just wasn't true with the people we were working with.

Emma's progress really gave us hope. Our case worker was always commenting to me that I had a great attitude. I supposed my attitude was good because I knew our girls would be free of this affliction in the Celestial Kingdom. I also knew that this was just a part of the test of this world and all I needed to do was the best I could.

I was nagged with interest in the factors that might be causing this epidemic. By this time, I knew far too many autistic children. There were four under the age of fourteen in our ward alone, and it looked like there would be three more diagnosed within the year.

When I was a child I don't remember any children in my ward who were autistic. There seemed to be physical symptoms that went largely untreated because the disability was all shrouded in a mystery called autism. Emma had allergies and dark, puffy bags under her eyes all the time. She had always had loose bowel movements, which I found to be disturbing. Essentially, I wanted to address these physical problems just as aggressively as we were addressing her educational needs. I began a search on the internet and in books. I looked into the GF/CF (gluten free/casein free) diet which parents have claimed helped alleviate many symptoms. I went to a class on diet and found out that there were theories about something called a "leaky gut," that is to blame for the autistic symptoms. This notion seemed incomplete to me, but I thought the idea was a place to start.

We took Emma off milk products first, since I had already suspected that Emma might be allergic to dairy products. We began this treatment a month before we started DTT, and the next day Emma started to sing. Her good mood seemed too soon to be related to milk. Ridding her body of milk should have taken at least seven days; so we thought her good mood was just interesting timing.

We continued with the milk elimination for three months. As Thanksgiving approached, we became more lax on the whole CF program. We couldn't tell if the diet was making any difference, so we just stopped. The teacher began noting that Emma wasn't her old self. She had gotten really quiet and wasn't singing anymore. We'd seen her go through lots of stages; so rather than blame the milk, we just figured her behavior was a stage.

Next I began researching the DAN (Defeat Autism Now) protocol. This program sounded promising. The doctors involved in the program were meeting yearly at a conference to discuss the possible treatments. They'd come up with a few things that sounded very proactive. One was called chelation, where they remove the heavy metals, particularly mercury, from the system. Now, mercury is very controversial; it can come from immunizations or tooth-fillings in the child or from the mother during pregnancy. This debate continues on in Congress and among doctors all over the world. Chelation itself has stirred some controversy because it's believed that in the process of chelating, the patient may have to endure the contamination all over again as the metals leave the tissues and flow back through the system. This method concerned our pediatrician; and his misgivings made some sense to me; so that wasn't the route for us— even though a local mother told of this treatment's having helped her son immensely.

Another thing these DAN doctors are doing is injecting a hormone called secretin. This treatment sounded interesting, but the doctors weren't really sure from a scientific standpoint why it worked. Still, a woman I exchanged e-mails with claimed her son was doing very well because of secretin. I wasn't ready to put much hope in something this unproven, so my search continued.

One day I received an e-mail from the same mother who told me about secretin. She told me about a doctor in California named Dr. Goldberg whom I might be interested in. She said she'd see him if she were closer (and if he didn't dislike secretin so much). He was treating children for a condition called Neuro-Immune Dysfunction Syndrome (NIDS). She gave me his website address so I could check into it. There I found an explanation that seemed to mesh with things I already was beginning to believe. Namely, I was thinking that this disfunction might be related to the immune system and how our bodies deal with viruses and environmental elements. Now, I didn't come to this idea out of the blue. For years our family had been battling some auto-immune related conditions. When Jeanette, our second daughter, was diagnosed with Graves' disease, the endocrinologist indicated that the disease seemed to run in families—even though it didn't seem to be genetic. Autism seemed to work the same way.

My grandmother had had Graves' disease and so did several of my cousins. Conversely, other members of the family (including me) were affected by the opposite condition, called Hashimoto's Thyroiditis (hypothyroidism). Interestingly, we had the same antibodies in our system. Our thyroids appeared to be responding to an auto-immune response.

Now, I had no idea why I thought this bit of information and autism had anything to do with one another, but the correlation just seemed logical. When I read from the NIDS website that there seemed to be a link between autism and conditions such as asthma, thyroid disorders, and certain viral conditions, something in my brain seemed to click. The supposition was that this wasn't some mysterious neurological condition, but rather an auto-immune system run amok and attacking the brain. The proposition tied into the "leaky-gut" theory showing how that could be a symptom of this auto-immune condition.

For the first time, my skeptical mind began to envision a medical direction for our daughter. We prayed to be directed beyond our ability to understand. We asked that we not be misled by charismatic individuals "promising the moon." We weren't really in a position to undergo an expensive medical path. I was sure that the cost would be prohibitive to see this particular doctor and that would be the end of the issue. I called the office and was told that he was only contracted with two insurance companies. What chance would we have that one would be ours? We didn't have the most common coverage. But, to my surprise, ours was on his list. That meant we would pay only $15 for our visits. I took this as an answer to my prayer, and we took the next available appointment, which was six months later.

As the appointment date neared, we were told by Dr. Goldberg's office that Emma should go back on the CF diet. We weren't thrilled. It was so nice not to worry about it. Only a few days after we eliminated milk products again, we got a note from Emma's teacher saying that we had our "old" Emma back. Since this was the only change we'd made, I began to connect the picture here. Emma really did have a negative reaction to milk. Her allergy wasn't so huge that we were afraid to give her milk, but it was big enough to be noticeable. That was the end of milk for Emma; although, I'll admit she has had an occasional treat of pizza, which was also on the negative list.

Emma didn't really fit the profile of the patients who could be most helped by Dr. Goldberg. He had his greatest success with children that clearly regressed into autism. Emma seemed always to be this way. We ran all the blood work he requested anyway. I asked our pediatrician what he thought of this NIDS theory. He had been very skeptical of the mercury-poisoning theory and the secretin treatment. He hadn't seen a lot of success when kids were on the GF/CF diet. He wasn't sure about the MMR theory, either.

I thought there was validity in all of these ideas, but, where NIDS was concerned, he said that this doctor seemed to be using solid, scientific studies; there wasn't much he could dispute. He also had another patient seeing Dr. Goldberg, and this child was the only one he thought had been helped by medical intervention He proceeded with ordering all the tests. [I'll never know if he thinks I'm a complete "nutcase"; but, so far, he's been respectful of my quest, as long as we continue DTT. That method is the only thing he really has any confidence in.]

Our visit with Dr. Goldberg was quite an experience. He spent over an hour with us, going over Emma's history and test results thoroughly. He confessed that Emma wasn't a clear case of NIDS. She only had slight abnormalities in her bloodwork, but, he wanted to treat her for these issues and see if we could get them straightened out. Maybe, clearing these things up would help Emma connect more to the world. He started her on an antiviral drug to stabilize her immune system. At the same time, he had us start giving her iron supplements, because she was anemic. Now, Emma had had her blood checked several times before for anemia. No doctor had ever taken her low count very seriously. They seemed to figure poor absorption was common in autism. Dr. Goldberg didn't take anything for granted.

Within days of giving Emma extra iron, she was eating foods she'd refused before. She ate more meat and even gave vegetables another chance. It was wonderful to see. We couldn't tell so easily the effects of the antivirals; that would be more evident from her bloodwork at the next visit. We also had her checked for allergies and found that she was, in fact, allergic to milk. The doctor also had us limit her whole-wheat consumption. After a few weeks he had us add an anti-fungal medication. This treatment was to stop her loose bowel movements. There is also a belief that autistic children have internal yeast problems in general. In a strange twist, my brother had been battling chronic hives for three years. The doctors only treated his symptoms with mega-doses of Allegra. I mentioned Emma's treatment for yeast; and the next thing I knew, my brother's hives were diagnosed as a result of an internal yeast infection. Yeast may be the plague of our day.

In January, Emma was supposed to be moved up to the Sunbeam class. The primary presidency was a bit concerned about how to accommodate her. I got some great ideas from the LDS_Autism e-mail list, including having a shadow person assigned to help her out. When the presidency met with me I proposed this idea. They expressed that they had been thinking the same thing. They wanted me to give input about who should be called to do this. Their first thought was to have Lila do it, since she was so good with Emma; but, maybe Lila needed to be somewhere else in the ward. All prayers led back to Lila. I told them that I trusted that they would work it out and that they could ask Lila to help out until they made their decision. So, we started the year with Lila being Emma's shadow. I was going to make a little booklet with cues to clue Emma in to what was happening; but, with Lila there, the booklet wasn't necessary. She pointed things out to Emma and helped her know what was going on. I don't quite know how Lila helped Emma accomplish the transition, since Emma still didn't understand so much; but at least, Emma seemed comforted. We were blessed that Emma tried to imitate the other children. Within a few months, Lila was more of an assistant to the teacher with all of the children. Emma no longer needed such personal attention. She had learned the order of things and tried to participate, which was wonderful to see.

Emma began having fewer tantrums and seemed to feel better. In my memory she seemed like she'd felt sick all along. At the end of Emma's first year in preschool, we met with her school psychologist, the administrator, and her teacher for the yearly IEP (individual education plan) meeting. The most memorable statement from that meeting was when the psychologist said that Emma was not the same little girl that started the year.

At the beginning of Emma's second year of preschool, the comment was that Emma wasn't "your typical autistic child." Granted, there is no typical autistic child. I take this to mean that Emma is being blessed with tremendous progress. Maybe to get professionals to see the possibilities. Maybe because we're going to find the answer to this mystery someday. Maybe just because it was the direction her life was supposed to take. Maybe she is autistic to point the direction for Megan's help.

I don't know all the reasons why these things happen, but I do know that autism will unlock the meaning of life for many people. To see, first hand, the delicacy of reality helps push out all the things that aren't really pertinent.

Chapter Five

"Where There is Great Love...."
Matthew, age 6
by Kathy Weatherford

Kathy Weatherford has been married for nearly 14 years to a very musical guy who is a wonderful husband and father, and she is "Mommy" to 4 great children. She wound up with a degree in Elementary/Early Childhood Education from BYU and taught kindergarten for a short time. She always wanted to write more, but didn't ever expect autism to be the subject! In her spare time (what?!) she likes to craft and decorate cakes and bake. Matt was diagnosed with autistic spectrum disorder at the age of 3 years 3 months.

My husband and I are sometimes told, "I really admire you for being the parent of an autistic child," or "You're doing such a great job with Matt—he's really progressing," or even, "You must really have been great spirits for Heavenly Father to have entrusted you with such a 'special' child!" We don't usually feel like we are doing a particularly great job parenting, and we certainly don't feel like we are anything special! Much of the time we only feel we aren't doing nearly enough for any of our four wonderful children. "Believe me," I want to reply, "I wasn't given this job because of some Heavenly Qualifying Exam, and I really don't possess any fabulous parenting skills that you should stand in awe of." I fuss at my kids all too frequently, as they would certainly tell you if you asked (please don't). I spend many days in tears because of the frustrations of trying to be a good parent. Yes, I am "blessed" to have a particularly urgent need for patience, but that doesn't mean I have mastered the skill. When friends talk to me, I am much more comfortable having them ask how I am holding up under the pressure instead of telling me that I am holding up so well. It helps me if they assume I need sympathy and understanding rather than feeling they need to cheer me up. Not that comments designed to help me see the good aren't welcome, but if they don't come with a dose of sympathy, they may sound more like a censure for my grief or guilt.

Just a couple of weeks after our third child, Matt, had been diagnosed with autism, I went to a party. I didn't feel much like partying (besides the impact of the diagnosis, I was two months' pregnant with our fourth);

but this was one of those parties where a friend was trying to get her home business off the ground, and I wanted to be supportive. So I went, knowing I would have to take Matt with me. As he started zipping around the room, dumping out baskets of books and toys without taking a second look or playing with any of them, I explained to my friends that his behavior had a reason—Matt had just been diagnosed with autism. One of the ladies encouragingly replied, "At least you can be glad he isn't sitting in a corner banging his head against the wall."

I'm sure my friend was trying to help me see the bright side and to be grateful for the blessings I did have. After all, we know many families with a child whose autism is more severe than Matt's, so in that way we really are blessed. Still, to us, no matter how much worse it "could be," that knowledge did not alleviate our very real and deep grief. We found that, all too frequently, friends and family were inclined not to take either our sadness or the diagnosis very seriously, since the little bit of Matt that they saw wasn't really the whole picture. Understanding autism involves so much more than just understanding the tidbits people hear about it (if they have even heard about it!). People insisted that he must only be "mildly" autistic. (In fact, although he isn't severely autistic, his isn't a mild condition, either. He is not what some refer to as "high functioning," since he doesn't "function" well in society yet, without a great deal of support.)

The comment about Matt's not sitting in a corner haunted me for several months. The sister who made the remark is very spiritual and has a really good understanding of the gospel. Was I really being an ungrateful daughter of God to grieve over having a son who might never be baptized, serve a mission, or even be able to speak an entire sentence—a son who would likely never be close to us in the same way our other kids were? Was my pain really ingratitude? Was it selfish to grieve for the loss of our son's "normal" adulthood and the realization that he might never even understand what he was missing? Ingratitude or just plain helplessness— I was feeling grief as well as confusion as to what I should do. I had joined the ranks of mothers who have a child with a disability, and I simply didn't know what I should think and feel. I wasn't bitter, but I also wasn't ready to believe that this could be a blessing.

From my college days, I would later remember an incident that illustrates the "be careful what you ask for" principle. At the time I just thought I was commenting on a minor career direction; but looking back, my comment seemed oddly momentous, somehow defining my life in a way

I hadn't intended. My choice to do a double major in Early Childhood/ Elementary Education had nothing to do with "getting my M.R.S. Degree." I really loved teaching children and wanted to be involved in a meaningful way in their lives. My coursework was exciting and fun for me; and when it came time to do the unit in Special Education, I studied with interest many types of disabilities. (It is perhaps interesting to note that I do not remember autism as something I studied; rather, I remember going to hear Kim Peek, the autistic savant who inspired the movie "Rain Man," address the students in the Education Department.) Part of that class involved volunteering for a few hours each week at the special needs school a few blocks from BYU. The work was fascinating, but really difficult, and I soon began to feel discouraged. Working with special needs kids was so exhausting, and sometimes I felt there was very little to show for it. Cheering a child for taking just one step wasn't enough to fill the holes in that child's life. They were just missing so much, and my heart often ached for those kids. My good friend, who was nearly done with her degree in Special Education, said, "Why not get your degree in Special Ed.? You would be great in that field!" I replied that she must be someone with an amazing level of patience to work with kids like that. "I just don't have what it takes to work with these kids all the time!" I told Carrie. "I get too frustrated waiting for those 'small miracles' and just wanting things to get better—now! I don't have the patience for that kind of work—I'd rather teach in a 'regular' kindergarten." And so I did.

Fast forward about nine years. Stephen and I had a beautiful five-year-old girl, a busy almost-two-year-old boy, and a brand-new baby boy. Born on the Fourth of July, we said he was our "Yankee Doodle Dandy," and sang that song to him frequently. He was beautiful, the product of an uncomplicated pregnancy and a slightly complicated delivery (my first non-Caesarian childbirth). As he grew, he did all kinds of cute things, like responding with wild giggles to the entertainment the older kids provided. Shortly after his first birthday, he surprised us by "singing" a song the older kids were singing. They had made up lyrics to "My Bonny Lies over the Ocean" using "brother" instead of "bonny." Matt would sing, "Ba, ba! Ba, Ba! Ba ba ba..." for the chorus, but the amazing thing was that he was actually on key. Anyone within hearing range would say, "Wow, he is really musical! I can tell exactly what tune he's singing! And he's only one year old!" By eighteen months, however, Matt still wasn't saying any real words, just echoing a few words and sentences. With my educational background, I told myself he was still right on target.

Lots of kids use what is called "parroting" to learn language, I reasoned. Developmentally, repeating what he had heard wasn't so unusual. Besides, it was really cute to hear him ask, "Are you finished?" when he wanted to get out of the high chair after a meal. Still, it was a little odd that he would stay quietly in that high chair for countless minutes after the meal just playing silently with a fork or a piece of food. We figured he was one of those really quiet children; and we actually were glad we didn't have to rush to get him out, since we were able to get more done right after the meal while he seemed amused.

About this time, Matt also began to exhibit really strange play skills—or, more accurately, a lack of play skills. He would run around the house dumping all the little toys out of their bins or boxes—not using them, just dumping them. He would look at things intently, turning them over and over in his little hands and putting them right up close to his face, but he would never play with them the way the other kids did. Of course, none of my kids had been exactly typical in play skills. Born with big imaginations, they never used blocks to build. Instead, blocks were candies on a tray, groceries in a store, or cars, or people, or just about anything. So in this respect, Matt's lack of play skills made sense, but the energy level he displayed with these habits was wearing me out. He would climb and run and get into things from morning 'til night, reminding me of a quote I saw at my friend's house: "A mother of boys has to work from son-up to son-down."

I was feeling like things were a little out of control, however, when I couldn't even use the bathroom without the house looking like "Hurricane Matt" had just blown through. Once at choir practice, a friend looked at me and said, "Is he like this ALL the time?" When I said, "Pretty much," she commented that I must be exhausted. I was. An observer might view him as hyperactive as they watched him repeatedly get into things, dump things out, and take things apart. I became the "Queen of Superglue" and an expert at videotape repair too, since videos were about the only way we could get five or ten minutes of peace at our house.

I remember a visit to Stephen's parents' home when his dad asked us, "Does Matt ever do anything besides watch videos? Doesn't he ever play with toys?" We tried to explain, but since we didn't understand his behavior ourselves, we felt at a loss to share with anyone else what our lives were like. I knew my father-in-law wasn't being critical, just genuinely puzzled by Matt's behavior; but I projected my feelings of inadequacy as a parent into my interpretation of his words. I internalized the criticism as "You let him watch too much TV!" even though I am sure that wasn't Dad's intention. I began to feel as though we really were strange and different from everyone else—and somehow incapable of doing the parenting thing the way it should be done (the way normal people parented!).

Another oddity was that Matt almost never slept through the night. His frequent awakenings and occasional super-early rising times really seemed unexplainable. (Have you ever had a child get up for the day at 3:30 am and sing or laugh uncontrollably for hours, only to fall asleep at 9:00 o'clock when the day is just getting going? It's not fun.) He still does that fairly often, but at that time we didn't know that sleeplessness is pretty typical for kids with autism. Everything I read in the child development books said that kids needed ten hours or more of sleep per night, so I really wondered how on earth Matt was growing properly.

The most frightening development for us, however, was his tantrums. When Matt was two, he was acting like a typical "terrible twos" child, but with one unnerving twist: he would stand up, stiffen, and throw himself backward, maintaining the stiff posture all the way to the floor. If he happened to be on a hard surface like the kitchen floor, he would then cry harder because he was hurt. Since we felt there might be real danger of serious head injury, we were very reluctant to use what we considered the optimal parenting skill in tantrum situations: walk away and wait for the child to get over it. However, since this was the only thing we felt certain would work, we cautiously withdrew our attention from Matt during the tantrum and waited for him to calm down so we could talk about it. To our distress, not only did this not work, but Matt's tantrums were increasing, not just in frequency, but in intensity and length as well. He could cry for more than 20 minutes, screaming and thrashing on the floor. I couldn't imagine why he wasn't quitting the behavior, when it was only hurting him.

We began to worry constantly that he would give himself a concussion. When I took Matt in for a well-baby check, the doctor asked about any concerns we had. I brought up the tantrums and their intensity; and he, looking at me in apparent seriousness, asked why Matt had tantrums. I thought to myself, "Is this guy for real? He must not have any kids." All kids have tantrums sometimes; it was just the intensity I was questioning. He reassured me that Matt wouldn't do any real damage to himself, that if it really hurt, he would stop. I wasn't sure I believed that. Matt was crying harder and longer than I had ever seen a child cry, and the collection of knots on his head was continuous.

One experience that really illustrates our frustration happened at Costco. I dared to brave taking all three kids there one day (a decision which some would say was a little over-ambitious in itself), hoping to simply grab the few items on my list and go. Matt had just turned three; and I knew he could be "a real handful" when shopping, so we had invested in a harness device with plastic hooks to attach to the shopping cart so he couldn't stand up. (Matt is the only one of my children who actually fell out of a shopping cart, headfirst, onto cement flooring no less, so I wasn't taking any chances.) Matt hated being restrained, and we always had a huge wrestling match to put the harness on. While my two older children wandered around with the gimmies," Matt threw a monstrous tantrum and actually snapped the big plastic hooks right in two. I could feel my face getting hot and tears pricking my eyes and decided then and there that I must be the world's most inept parent. We had used every good parenting technique we could and still couldn't manage, or explain, these violent tantrums. What I didn't know was that articles like "Parenting the Strong-Willed Child" weren't meant to handle someone with autism.

When a lady approached me to offer help, I turned away, embarrassed beyond belief and mumbling that I would cope and thanks for offering. All the time I was collecting the big kids, I was fighting back tears, wondering, "Why are we failing at parenting so miserably? My other children are pretty well behaved, and I have been using the same basic techniques for this one. What is wrong with us?"

To complicate things even further, there were lots of behaviors that fooled us into thinking Matt was extremely gifted. He picked up the amazing habit of pointing to letters and identifying them out loud. One day on my bed, he was saying letters: "B, R, I, pause...H, A, M, Y, O, U, N, pause...U, N, I, V..." I did a double take when I realized he was spelling Brigham Young University from the logo on my tote bag, but didn't know the letter "g." Matt was only 18 months old, and I couldn't believe he could name all those letters! I figured then and there we were rearing a genius child! He sang well, and on key. He could recognize all his videos from text labels only, no pictures. He memorized huge scenes from his favorite videos and could communicate his thoughts using dialogue from these scenes. Little did I know that this memorization/parroting skill signaled a problem, not simply being gifted.

Over the course of the next several months, until he was about two and a half, we had some odd experiences that made us seriously begin to wonder about our Matt's development. The parroting got worse—he never said anything using original language. Matt also seemed increasingly disconnected from us. I had his hearing tested a couple of times and was told it was fine Actually, I knew it was okay because I could whisper the word "cookie" when he was two rooms away and he would come running. It was decidedly peculiar, though, that he couldn't seem to hear if I called his name aloud just four feet away. Getting his attention was nearly impossible. I had heard the jokes about the "selective deafness" of children when they were listening to their parents, but this was certainly the worst case I had ever seen.

My calling at the time was Relief Society secretary, and one of my good friends in the presidency mentioned Asperger's Syndrome (which is a condition on the autistic spectrum), so I read a bit about it. Stephen and I decided Asperger's couldn't possibly be what we were dealing with, yet we still recognized some of the pieces of our puzzle. Apparently Asperger's kids had language that developed just fine, and I knew Matt didn't have that. He did allow cuddling and he didn't have too many glaring sensory issues, so we felt something on the autism spectrum just didn't make sense. Some of Matt's most autistic behaviors, manifested in recent years, were also there when he was younger. They were just not so glaringly obvious in a two-year-old, since they might just have been little bits of lingering babyhood. We had a hard time judging because the development of our two older kids had differed greatly, yet still had been within the broad range of typical. I was convinced that since I had a degree in child development, I wasn't going to be one of those "paranoid parents" who jumped on any seeming abnormality and made a huge issue of it. We were taught in school that all children develop at different rates and that parents just need to relax, have patience, and not worry if their child doesn't do everything right on schedule. Stephen and I decided that we would wait until Matt turned three and then talk to our family doctor if things still seemed unusual.

About two months before Matt's third birthday, our parental instincts overtook our intellectual reasoning. We called our doctor who, thank heavens, felt enough confidence in us to not dismiss our concern. I said I felt that something was not right about Matt's development. I laid out my concerns in a concise list: not much language, only echoing; not playing with toys; not attending to his name; and the tantrums (Oh yes, the tantrums!). Our doctor arranged for us to see specialists at a local speech, language, and learning center. The evaluator there mentioned Pervasive Developmental Disorder (PDD, which is the broader category that autistic spectrum disorder falls under) as a possibility, but said she wasn't the one with the qualifications to diagnose that, and that it was best diagnosed later on. (The current thinking is that PDD can and should be diagnosed before two years of age and as early as you can catch the signs. Studies have been done on babies' first birthday party videos, and experienced researchers can pick out children with autism quite accurately, when versed in what signs to look for.) We wished later that she had sent us straight to a neurologist.

We found out later how important knowing early can be for these kids—every day counts! We began reading about autism and other Pervasive Developmental Disorders, but we still were confused by the myths: "Autistic children aren't affectionate and don't like to be touched." We knew that wasn't true of Matt, since he always came to me to be held and was even nearly obsessed by playing with my hair. In fact, one of his first attempts at a sentence of original language was (talking to me), "Oh, you're my hair!" Other myths were, "Autistic children don't speak." We heard that one everywhere, but Matt spoke—a lot. He repeated everything he heard, and could recite word for word all those scenes from Sesame Street and Blue's Clues videos. He learned songs from his favorite CD's with ease—so he couldn't be autistic, right? But he used those video conversations and songs to communicate, never using his own words. Was he gifted or not? Many of the portents of something serious were there. He couldn't carry on a conversation, never pointed, didn't pretend, or play with toys. He never tried to show us anything that interested him. He never vied for attention with his siblings—perhaps one of the strangest things of all!

A good speech pathologist from Speech, Language, and Learning began seeing Matt, and after a few months, she sent us to the neurologist. He explained that autism is diagnosed very subjectively. We had been requested to fill out many pages of questions about Matt and his development, everything from my pregnancy with Matt, to family history, to what Matt eats, and at what age he met all the typical milestones of babyhood. That was especially hard, since he was my third child, and the baby book wasn't as perfectly kept as I would have liked! The papers took me hours to complete, and I didn't know what they would tell anyone when I was finished. The neurologist spent a few minutes observing Matt. He asked what seemed to us like endless questions, poring over all that paperwork. His diagnosis was Autistic Spectrum Disorder. As prepared as we felt we had been to hear this, since we had been suspecting it for a while, it felt like it sort of slammed into our souls when we actually had it from the official source. I was kind of numb for a few days, and then I knew we had to move fast to do something. I didn't do much crying and grieving right then. For me, this has been a continual process of crying and grieving every so often. Whenever I spend time around kids of his age and younger who communicate effortlessly, I might come out crying. The Christmas before the diagnosis, visiting Stephen's family was a particularly difficult ordeal. Matt's younger cousin Noah was very good with language and very precocious and social. As I watched that darling little boy play and talk with all the cousins and saw my own darling little boy sitting over in a corner, not responding to any friendly overtures from the family (just playing oddly with objects and watching videos), I kept trying to hide my tears.

About one month before the diagnosis, we discovered that I was expecting our "newest model," the fourth child in our family. Having a new baby gave us something new to worry about; we soon found as we began to read statistics on autism in families that already have a child with autism. The statistics of having a child with autism in the first place have most recently been quoted as somewhere between 1 in 250 to 1 in 500 children, but if you already have one on the spectrum, the odds are something like 10 to 20 times greater that your other children will be on the spectrum. Personally, I have come across many families who have more than one child on the spectrum, some having kids all over the spectrum from mild to severe. We were from that moment on concerned about out next child's development. A friend of mine who has three kids, with her middle one having Down's Syndrome, was telling me what a wonderful thing having a younger typically developing sibling has been for her Down's child. She told me how the younger one pushes the older one to do the things he is doing. The older one says, "Well, if my little brother can do it. . . ."

We are hoping that will happen for Matt, as we see David already at age 18 months doing things that Matt struggles with. We hope and pray that autism has passed him by, as it seems to have.

The diagnosis sent us riding a whirlwind of reading, studying, joining internet list groups to talk to other parents, and generally trying to learn everything we could about autism. The neurologist gave us a sheaf of papers with contact information for a couple of organizations, and a booklist. Before we left, he gave us the advice that I believe has "saved" us. He told us that we would hear about and possibly try many things to help with Matt's autism. He said there were all kinds of interventions out there, but only one had a proven track record of empirical evidence in helping kids with autism to progress. Lots of studies out there showed that ABA, or Applied Behavioral Analysis, was the best way to get children with autism on the learning track. He showed us a rather large book about behavioral interventions for young children with autism that was a super resource for learning about ABA and getting started. We contacted Families for Effective Autism Treatment, Washington Chapter (FEAT-WA) and heard all about getting started with an ABA program. We learned we needed a "consultant," a professional who would write and coordinate Matt's program for us, and therapists to carry out the program. Then we began the work of calling the local organizations that do this, and the frustrations of finding waiting lists of indeterminate length for all of them. Since we had been told with much emphasis by many people that every day counted and that we had to get going on intervention, we were feeling more stressed by the day. Meanwhile, I was spending hours every day phoning people and places, reading enormous amounts of information about autism, and especially reading about ABA and all the studies. It was wonderful reading, since I finally was beginning to understand that all of the odd behaviors and problems I saw in Matt had a reason—a connection with something real and recognized. But the more I read, the more I knew that ABA was what Matt needed; and as the days slipped by, I had no idea how we were going to get there. We did lots of praying, and I made an appointment to talk to a private consultant who didn't have a waiting list. Then I got a phone call that would change our lives.

FEAT had set me up with a mentor, a lady who had an autistic child a few years older than mine, who had gone through countless interventions and work, and who was really well informed about autism and the journey we were just starting. As we talked, she told me about this wonderful ABA consultant who had administered her child's program. This family had literally picked up and moved to Oregon for a year just to work with this consultant. She gave me a glowing report about how great he was and what an excellent job he had done with her child. He had just moved here to Washington to start his own consulting organization, Lodestar Development, Inc. Our mentor said that Lodestar was just getting going here and probably didn't have a waiting list. That was so exciting to hear that the second I finished with her, I got on the phone and made an appointment with Lodestar right away. In a short time, I actually had two appointments with consultants who didn't have waiting lists! So now our prayers turned in the direction of helping us choose what was right for Matt.

We interviewed the first consultant on our list, and I was pleased with what I heard, but not entirely confident that she was the one to best serve Matt. A few nights later, we had our first consultation with David Cole. Having a thorough background in child development, I needed only about 10 minutes to see that this guy really knew his stuff. After just one visit, not only was he teaching us about autism, but—even more than that—he was figuring out our son for us. His credentials were impressive, but I might have taken a chance on him even without them, because I could see that he really knew how to do something that was above and beyond plain ABA as I had read about it in the books. And he loved and cared about children. We also met his fiancée soon after that, and she was also very talented, and experienced in her own areas of providing for these children both in school settings and in home therapy sessions. We felt so right about hiring Lodestar, and we have never regretted it, in so many ways.

Earlier in the year, Stephen and I had had some of his corporate stock options come up, and we had talked about investing the money but had not gotten around to it. We now found out how much a good ABA program costs and that insurance did not cover it, since it is behavioral therapy and not traditional speech or occupational therapy. We now knew why we had not "gotten around" to investing that money. We knew it would be invested in a way we could not have imagined. Matt's program costs approximately $25,000 per year. We know people who have second-mortgaged their homes or who have gone into other forms of debt to get this program for their kids. We have been blessed not to have to, at least not yet! We have friends who have cut the costs down by trying to do more of it themselves, or by training and hiring young women from their ward to do most of the work. I know I personally couldn't have brought Matt anywhere near as far as he has come, without David as our guide.

We soon realized that no one we knew understood the seriousness of what we were experiencing. Our families didn't realize; our friends didn't understand; our ward family didn't know. Our little ones usually look "normal" and are often quiet and sort of walled off from the world. While people recognize a behavior problem when it jumps up and knocks them down (maybe literally!), they don't often realize that a quiet, self-absorbed child who doesn't talk a lot (which means he doesn't talk out of turn) could be a child unable to understand language and the world around him. People would give back to us the myths we had debunked with our research; and the myths were just as pervasive as our child's problem.

"Oh, Matt talks, though. He must just be very mildly autistic." I would want to shout in their faces, "But have you listened to what he says?" They would also say they saw him show affection, or sitting quietly, saying anything they could think of to make it seem like things must not be as bad as we thought. It seemed no one wanted to accept the diagnosis as it stood. We struggled to make people see the lifelong nature of what we are dealing with; and even today we continue to get so many comments about how much better he is (which is true) and how he must be just about to overcome the problem. I remember my visiting teacher coming to visit and watching Matt have a real meltdown about something I had tried to explain to him he could not do, but he still wanted to. His frustration at not understanding the subtleties of language often caused him to cry and scream on the floor, and I must admit that when you see an older child do that, it is very disconcerting. She commented to me later that what she saw when visiting me at home gave her a much better understanding of what we were dealing with. She basically said that what everyone saw at church was an incomplete picture, and that she was glad of the chance to realize what the troubles were more completely. That conversation made me realize the great need to educate people around Matt about autism. I was particularly touched by a talk I heard in our ward one Sunday about a man who had been coaching youth and had terrible behavior problems with one of his young athletes—only to discover later that the young man suffered from Tourette's Syndrome. He said in his talk that he could have been so much more effective as this boy's coach if he had known about the problem and how to deal with it, but that the parents of the boy were trying not to talk much about their son's problem. That talk made me understand what I had to do.

We needed to help our ward family understand what was going on. We knew that bringing up Matt would take lots of help, love, encouragement, and support from everyone around us. I had been pondering how much help I felt I needed. How often I tried to explain to people what autism is and what we do about it. I was so tired of trying to keep explaining; but I knew if our ward family was ever going to understand Matt and his behaviors and needs, I was going to have to keep explaining for a long time!

Autism is so generally misunderstood. All most people know is what is portrayed in the movies and media (which only present a few facets of the problem). I definitely wanted to do this explaining for our family's sake, but it was disheartening having to explain over and over to all the people individually. One day in ward council meeting (I was the activities committee chairman at the time) we were discussing the needs of ward members and how activities could meet those needs. I suddenly blurted out that it would be good to have a night where we could get together everyone in the ward—including the people who currently work with Matt in nursery and Primary, the bishopric, and others who were curious—and teach them about autism. I then became embarrassed (was everyone wondering, "What is she thinking?") and said something like, "Of course, Bishop, only if you think that would be appropriate." Then I shut up quickly. I think I was holding my breath while I watched the Bishop think a second, then he said he thought it would be very appropriate. I said it could be done in our home, but he assigned the Relief Society to sponsor it (though I specifically invited Matt's Primary leaders) The Relief Society helped publicize it, and we lined up the Relief Society room for the event. They called it a "Special" Enrichment Night, and we invited the whole ward. We invited the youth, especially those who might baby-sit for our family, and everyone else we could think of. I knew it would be much more effective if I was not the one speaking, since people tend to listen when they have an expert in front of them—especially if that expert is an interesting speaker! We told our consultant David that we would love to hire him for the evening to do this presentation, and he said that he would be happy to do it for free, because raising autism awareness in the community was important to him. Later, we realized how many of his hours were spent on that presentation, and we were so grateful to him for spending his time that has reaped many rewards for us.

That night was a turning point for us, in more ways than one. About twenty people showed up; more would have come had we not accidentally scheduled over a Cub Scout Pack Meeting and an orchestra rehearsal for a big stake concert! David gave us permission to tape the presentation and even to give copies to anyone we wanted, such as family and friends who couldn't be there. He spoke for around an hour and then opened the floor for questions. What happened then was another answer to prayer and a testimony of what can and should happen in any ward family that cares about each other. Not only were people really trying to understand and ask questions, but something that has been very helpful to us was born—

the "Matt Minute." One very enthusiastic brother in our ward asked the question, "I only see Matt for a few minutes between meetings on Sunday. What could I do, in just that short a time, to be helpful to him?" I said perhaps it would be a good time to work on social and language skills, such as eye contact, and how to respond to conversations and questions. I said I supposed that I could just tell people what Matt was currently working on, and they could ask a question that we had already helped him learn how to answer appropriately—sort of a planned conversation. That is a good way to help autistic kids learn to live with the world, by teaching them what they are likely to face and how to respond to it.

The sister who typed the program each week, who had worked with Matt in the children's class at Enrichment nights and had been so encouraging in all we did with Matt, said, "Maybe we could print a little paragraph in the bulletin, telling people what to ask Matt about this week and how they can help him work on this!" She cleared it with the bishop, and now, each week in our Sunday program our friends can read the "Matt Minute" and know what Matt is working on They can help him have short, successful, social conversations where he can work on eye contact and appropriate responses. It has been wonderful! Even a couple of teenage boys who don't know our family really well have come up to Matt and said, "Hi Matt, how are you doing?" With a shy smile, and a very wooden-sounding, "I'm good" (that's the only response he knows to that question), he answers them. We started with "What's your name?" "How old are you?" "What is your sister's name, [brother's name, and baby brother's name]?" Over and over we practice these things, until he can begin to answer more complicated things like, "What's your favorite food [video, song]?" "Where did you go on your trip? What did you see there?" For children with autism, practice makes perfect; and they never can stop practicing or they lose the skills they have.

That night, I finally recognized just how far Matt had come. David borrowed some video clips from us of Matt's third birthday, his fourth birthday, and recent clips of my playing with him. He had clips of when they first began to see him in an ABA program, and I realized then just how much ABA has blessed all of our lives, and not just Matt's. I was watching this montage of videos and remembering just how bad it had been before we knew what was wrong.

On Matt's third birthday, his cousins from Memphis were here as well as his brother and sister. In every clip, the kids were so excited they were dancing all around him, saying, "Oooh, Matt! Look at the present!

Come open this! You tear it like this, see?" They would practically shove the packages into his hands. He just wandered off, turning his back on everyone. He looked like he didn't even hear them! How strange, I thought, watching this. I didn't remember it being that bad. It's as if he is just in some kind of alternate universe, completely and sublimely unaware of everything going on around him—unknowing, uncaring. The next clips were of when David first worked with Matt. They were teaching him nouns, one word at a time. I had remembered that part well, a single noun with a picture to go with it. Learning word by word, having to make eye contact with the therapist to complete the drill. When he came to the section of the video that was Matt's fourth birthday, I was pulled up short. In just eight months, he had gone from learning single nouns to singing "Happy Birthday" to himself, asking me to put Elmo on his cake, counting the candles, and telling people—when asked—that he was four years old. When one of his therapists asked him the next day what he got for his birthday, he told her, "Fireworks!" (Being born on the Fourth of July, he must get pretty excited thinking all that stuff is for him!)

Since that time, I have watched Matt's fifth birthday tape. We were actually able to have a sort of conversation with him beforehand about what he wanted for his birthday. Of course, for an almost five-year-old, the conversation wasn't without peculiarities.... Me: "So, Matt. What do you want for your birthday?" Matt: "You can open presents on your birthday. Me: Yes, but what kind of present do you want for your birthday? Matt: Pink. Me: What kind of present? Matt: Blue. Purple. Me: Not what color it's wrapped in. What kind of toy do you want inside the package? Matt: Barney.

Later on in the conversation, he told me he was also interested in "Elmo guitar." This time, when he opened his packages, he would partially open one, peek through the wrapping paper, and say, with a very exaggeratedly excited voice (but basically appropriate!), "Ohhhhhh, it's a Barney Fishing game!" To our delight, he really enjoyed our singing to him, and he was able to tell people—when they asked later—what he got for his birthday. He really has come a long way. He is beginning to use more complex sentences. Many parts of speech still either don't make sense to him, or he is unable to use them appropriately; but, his skills get better all the time.

Attending our church meetings has come with unique difficulties, in spite of all the support of ward members. One meeting in particular stands out as example of some of these problems. We were late (as is often the case); Stephen was already there and playing the organ, so I had all four kids to tend. Being late, we weren't able to sit in our "usual" spot. We came in during the opening hymn, and when I started toward the other side of the chapel, Matt just collapsed to the floor, crying "NO! Sit THERE!" (pointing to the place we usually sat). I scooped Matt up, half-carrying, half-dragging him; and holding on to David, too, I headed to the chosen place. Then I suddenly heard the dead silence around me and realized that there was someone at the stand waiting to deliver the invocation. Everyone was waiting for me! Matt wasn't getting any quieter, so I turned right around and headed out. Between David trying to slip out of my arms to get down, and my carrying a bawling, squirming Matt, I barely made it out of the chapel without stumbling over my own heels. I sat in the foyer holding back the sobs. It is one thing to understand that autism is the problem, but sometimes living with it is another thing entirely. No fewer than three people sought me out after the service to tell me not to stress about it, that they understood, that no one blamed me, and so forth. One of my good friends even made me laugh by suggesting they rope off a pew for us that said on a nice brass plaque, "Reserved for the Weatherford Family."

There have been other needs and problems connected with church. Matt spent most of his Sunbeam year in the nursery since he was just getting good at handling the routine in there (and for a child with autism, routine is everything). We are very grateful to the loving Primary presidency and Nursery leaders who understood what he needed, and let this very tall child stay in the nursery with the little ones for so long. We parents of children with autism so badly need those loving leaders to be flexible and prayerful in their administration of the church programs, so we can feel a part of things. A lady just starting with our e-mail group broke all of our hearts with her statements about feeling that there was no place for her child at church, and so they were unable to attend church as a family. If there is one thing that we who understand the gospel should be champions at, it is making everyone know there is a place for them in our wards! We parents spend so much time advocating with the school systems to get the educational needs of our children met, and with the world in general, trying to help everyone understand our situations and our misunderstood children. We badly need to have ward leaders and members who will just love us enough to say to us, "I don't know how we will make this work, but we will find a way to help you be part of our ward!" As parents of these special kids, we still want to serve in our wards, but our resources of time and energy are few. Helping us to find extra support in teaching the gospel to our little ones, no matter how simple the lesson must be, is a strong testimony of the ward "family" and gives us the much needed break of serving someone other than our own families.

We are fortunate to have a Primary president who is committed to the teachings of the church about taking care of everyone in our ward family. This great lady has been Relief Society president and in the stake Relief Society, as well as being one of Matt's Nursery leaders at the time we got his diagnosis. She is firm like a rock and has insisted that helping Matt have a good church experience isn't just his family's responsibility, but hers, and his teacher's, and others' in the ward. She always greets Matt personally with a smile and feels bad when she can't. Our whole Primary presidency is incredibly supportive of us and our efforts, from using a picture schedule to help Matt see visually what is happening during Primary time, to encouraging the bishopric to call "shadows" for Matt, so we can attend our other meetings and hold callings while Matt has someone helping him with all the demands of Primary attendance.

Having others work with Matt has been a great blessing for us because it has allowed us to take a break from our responsibilities with Matt and to enjoy our own Sunday meetings more. We haven't realized until recently how desperately we need breaks from constantly being on-call, and how much we need the spiritual boost that our own meetings give us on Sunday. His shadow helps him focus on the action, stay seated, sing, and participate as best he can, though much of what he is hearing is like a foreign language to him, and he can only understand a word or two here and there. He can't understand concepts like repentance, faith, or even sharing, choosing the right, or following Jesus. Nearly all autistic children are extremely visual learners, and need to see pictures of concepts or see the action to understand it. That is why emotions and complex gospel concepts are so difficult for people with autism. Since they cannot see Jesus Christ, how can they know he is there?

Autism is truly terrifying for me still, even though generally I am better and better able to deal with the everyday effects. Autism cripples the ability to share thoughts; it cripples the ability to understand and express complex emotions. Matt has recently begun to express excitement and anticipation for some events, and the joy we find in his response is inexpressible. He is actually looking forward to Christmas this year, although like most five-year-olds he is most interested in what's in it for him! We don't care—we are starting to see what is going on inside that head of his, and we love seeing it!

I am a person for whom relationships have been the most important thing in my life. I like to be emotionally close to people, to know their feelings, thoughts, hopes and dreams, and to share mine. Really knowing people well—whether it is my husband, my children, the people who work with my kids, my friends, or anyone dear to me—is part and parcel of understanding them and loving them. With Matt, there is a huge wall and gap for this kind of relationship. I could tell you much of the time what my other kids love, what they are good at, what scares them, and often what they think about. We can't do that with Matt. He just isn't capable of the language to tell us that most of the time. Even the baby has more range of emotion than Matt does, and I continue to hope that this skill can be learned. Reading success stories of children who have recovered from autism with just a couple of years of ABA had built unrealistic hopes for quick improvement. We are still learning that the much-acclaimed success stories are the atypical cases and that most kids do not completely recover, although they can continue to improve. The process is more likely to take many years or even a lifetime, however. I keep telling myself that I can wait for it, but patience isn't my best virtue. My relationship with Matt builds in little bits and pieces, bright moments when I am least expecting anything of importance to happen. Suddenly he will look in my eyes and tell me something or invite me to laugh with him at something. Yes, I can wait for it!

As parents of typical kids, our worries about the future usually are things like, "Will they choose the right career? The right spouse? Will they stay strong in the gospel? Will they serve missions?" With Matt, our worries are much more basic, and frustrating: "Will my child be able to make friends? Can he understand the gospel? Will he ever be able to be baptized? Would he ever be able to marry? Parent a child?"

Parents of a child with autism have completely different sets of concerns. Right after the diagnosis, we asked our home teacher for blessings. We were feeling so unsettled and felt we needed the support. I was electrified to hear him tell me that Matt would overcome his autism and that he would serve a mission. He also reminded me, in the same blessing, that our time frame and the Lord's time frame are not the same and that we need to remember that. I cling to that blessing like the only buoy that keeps me afloat some days. I know the time will come, even if it's not at the usual time for things like that to happen. I often remind myself that Matt will be capable of understanding the gospel to the extent of being able to share it with others. That will be our own miracle, no matter on whose time schedule it occurs.

The blessings have been like the proverbial silver lining of the cloud—ever-present, but hidden until you look for them. Our older children are learning a level of compassion and tolerance that most kids never need to learn, and I am glad for their awareness. Amy, who is 10, had a young man in her fourth-grade gifted class who is autistic, and she was explaining to me how the other kids didn't know how to handle his outbursts and crying. She felt she was better equipped to understand him and was able to help explain a little to the others. Rob has had to grow up knowing that the brother who is closest to him in age is unable to play with him, unable to be that friend to him that he wishes for. He has been watching ABA sessions lately, trying to learn how to get Matt to play with him, to learn how to relate to him. Just this morning I watched Matt look at Rob over the Froot Loops and say, "Rob, be Cookie Monster." After giving him a very odd look, Rob just said, "OK," and started stuffing his mouth with cereal, making the appropriate Cookie Monster noises, and getting a huge giggle from Matt. Matt loved it, and said, "Rob, are you Cookie Monster?" It was good to see, since sometimes we have to get into Matt's world to bring him more into our world.

Other blessings are that I have been learning patience and learning to allow others the opportunity to serve me when sometimes I can't give back to them the way I want to be able to. I have learned to not let what others think, paralyze me and have learned to swallow back prideful feelings about having well-behaved children. I have been blessed beyond belief with caring people to help me with Matt; and although we have lots of stress in our family, we still love each other; and that love has been proved through uncomfortable circumstances. Through autism groups, we are blessed with new friends that we never would have known. I have been blessed to be able to put my education to work in ways I never would have conceived and to increase my learning continually in the field of autism. (We have joked amongst family that I might as well get my master's degree in autism research, since I have spent so many hours in that pursuit.)

An article by a parent of a child with autism asked the most breath-taking hypothetical question I have ever pondered in my life: "If there was a cure for autism that had no side-effects, and was proven safe, would you cure your child?" A few parents said that they believed that autism is who their child is; it is part of them, and they wouldn't take that away.

I don't feel that way. Although I do believe that some of these traits and abilities that he has are part of his personality, I believe that autism is something that stands as a barrier between Matt and his world. As for me, I know that Matt's spirit is there, capable of complex emotions and relationships. I think the "real" Matt wouldn't be bothered by these sensory and related issues—like being completely obsessed by having the left sock on before the right sock, or having to watching every video from the very beginning, including every preview and FBI warning screen. I believe that when Matt is resurrected he will be made whole, and this condition called autism will be dropped from his spirit, that he will be able to have relationships with us as our Heavenly Father intends all of us to relate to each other. And as for the blessing I received, I would hope that Matt will overcome his autism during his time here on earth and be able to serve a mission in his earthly lifetime. I have high hopes for him, even though I have to make adjustments to those hopes every so often. Two years ago I had hoped that by now (age five) he would be able to go to kindergarten without a shadow, and fit in. Now, I just hope we can get potty-training down before age six! But when I look at where Matt was and where he is now, I can't resist a smile at the realization that he is progressing one step at a time. I realize that I am learning to cheer for the small miracles, and that I can "work with special needs kids."

My Relief Society president frequently quotes the scripture from Alma 37:6, "By small and simple things are great things brought to pass." That could easily be the creed for ABA: that small and simple things bring about the great changes. But I also need the framed Willa Cather quote I got for Christmas from my husband—"Where there is great love there are always miracles." We have been given Matt, and we love him with a great love.

Chapter Six

Isaak, age 5
by Audra Jensen

I never thought I would meet a child in diapers who could read—let alone be called his mother. Then again, there have been a lot of things that have happened to me in the last few years that I might never have dreamed of. Never could I have imagined what changes would be wrought in my soul as I attempted to help my struggling child.

I was given a father's blessing soon after I found out I was pregnant with our first child. I was blessed with the strength I needed to grow strong and healthy in body. The blessing also said that the deficiencies that would occur in this child's growth would be overcome. But the pregnancy had no complications! In fact, I felt better when I was pregnant than I had ever felt before. During birth, however, there were complications; and Isaak was eventually brought into this world by emergency C-section. However, the child still had no noticeable problems. He was healthy and strong, especially considering that he was four weeks early. I was perplexed by the words in that blessing.

It's funny how sometimes life seems so perplexing—perhaps too often in my own life. I'll receive some personal guidance or words in a blessing that won't make sense until much later; or it might seem to make sense, but it won't be until some time later that the true meaning comes clear to me. How often I have sought out direction in my life, only to be given a puzzle to solve, a code to decipher. Then, when the answer becomes clear, I find that it was the journey from which I learned the most, not the answer.

Isaak was less than two years old when his sister was born. I still didn't know Isaak had autism, but I knew something was wrong. Little did I know what was to happen to him over the next few months. Nothing could have prepared me for it. That's why what happened that fateful evening of his sister's birth has taken on new meaning in the months (and now years) since.

I found myself in the same situation I had experienced two years earlier—having complications during labor, resulting in an emergency C-section. This time, though, the difficulty was much worse. By the time they began the operation, I felt as if I were "teetering on the edge." The doctors can say all they want that physically I was fine; deep-down, I knew something was not right. My life was in the Lord's hand—I knew that—and yet, I was frightened.

I was named after my maternal grandmother who had died just a few years before. I had been quite close to her in her later years. During that delicate operation, as I teetered on the edge of consciousness, I dreamt of her. She had a kind face and loving eyes. Our conversation was simple and her words were direct.

"You're okay. Everything is going to be fine."

I remember feeling relief. I knew she was right.

"Her name will be Audra."

We had chosen the name Rachel Margaret for our daughter—Rachel, because my husband and I couldn't agree on any other name, and Margaret after Dave's great-grandma and one of my good friends. We hadn't felt a strong connection to the name Rachel, but we hadn't come up with any other name that we could agree on. I wasn't surprised to hear that we had chosen an ill-fitting name. But Audra? I didn't want to give her the same name as mine. It was such an adult name for a baby.

"Audra? Do we have to name her Audra?" I asked my grandmother.

"Audra is her name," she said directly.

"What about her middle name—Margaret?" She told me that was fine.

"These are the two children you promised to take into your home. If you choose to have more, that's up to you; but these are the two you promised to have." She was very brief and straightforward, but her face was filled with love. I could feel it all around me. I remember thinking there were all sorts of questions I wanted to ask, but I couldn't think of any! Then she was gone.

I awoke again to the sounds of a newborn baby's cry. "You have your daughter," Dave whispered to me, tears in his eyes.

"Her name is Audra," I quietly returned to him.

I have often reflected on the words my grandmother left me with that fateful evening. "Everything's going to be fine." At the time, I was sure she was talking about the birth. As time went on, however, my mind often returned to that night. She was talking about more than the birth of my daughter.

My grandmother was preparing me. I had no way of knowing the challenges that lay ahead as I ventured to parent these two children. There were dark periods in those early years when I didn't know how I was going to make it through another day. I felt like a failure, like I could not possibly handle what the Lord thought I could. At the end of a day like that, I would collapse on my bed—physically, mentally, and spiritually drained. But, it was in those dark hours that I would reflect back on those words and remember that I had agreed to take on these challenges. I signed up for this life. Somehow, I knew I could do it; and I knew that these were special children that chose to come to my home—to be taught by me. I had a responsibility to them.

At the time of my daughter's birth, Isaak was nearly two years old. After appearing to be developing normally, he gradually began to be different from his peers. He became more socially aloof. He didn't have any useful language. His days were flooded with tantrums and rituals. He would stare at himself for long periods of time in a mirror, but he had little eye contact with others. He would line up plastic letters along the floor and crawl back and forth along the line, reciting the alphabet. He carried a book with him wherever he went. He didn't play with toys as other children did. All he wanted were those letters. If he didn't have one with him, he'd see one in his environment—he'd use his figures to make letters; he'd read the license plates as we walked through a parking lot; he'd watch "Wheel of Fortune" religiously in the evenings

His quirks were intriguing to everyone who knew him. How could a child, a near baby, seem so bright and yet struggle with some of the most basic milestones that children must pass? By the time he was two, he was reading, and his oddities were more evident than ever. We received the official diagnosis—autism and hyperlexia. He had significant delays in language, social, and behavior skills (autism) and yet had a keen intellect as evidenced in his early reading fascination (hyperlexia). I had no concept at the time how much our lives would be changed from that moment on. I had no idea how much I would come to rely on the Lord and learn to leave my troubles in His hands.

I knew at the moment Isaak received the diagnosis that I couldn't wait one day for him to "come out of it" on his own, like some people recommended to me. "Just give him time. Boys talk later than girls. Look how smart he is! What other two-year-old can read? He's just an active toddler. He'll be fine."

I heard these comments time and time again. However, I felt in my soul that this problem was something I had to attack, just as I would if he had been diagnosed with leukemia. I believed in him; I believed that, with hard work on his part, he could make the progress I knew he had in him. Once he received and I understood the diagnosis, I did my research. I found a program that would give him the best chance. This little two-year-old would be engaged in rigorous therapy from the moment he woke up to the moment he went to bed. He would have to learn how to talk, how to look at people, how to act, even how to play. Everything would have to be taught to him because he was not learning in any other way.

In the beginning, he had to be taught how to sit and attend to instruction. He did not like this. "Attending" went against everything natural in him. He would scream and resist even sitting directly across from someone. He would not look at them. He would not "tap table" when he was asked. All he would do was scream. In fact, in the first few months, that's almost all we heard. He was a fighter. Somehow, though, he knew that the instruction was for his own good. Yes, he would scream and protest almost every single session; yet during the day when he wasn't working, he'd take my hand and lead me up to the therapy room, as if to ask me to work. Then, gradually, he began to do more work and less resisting; and the gaps began to fill in.

Isn't that how it is in life? We scream and resist and protest at every hard thing we are asked to do. Yet somehow, deep down, we know the challenge is for our own good. We learn that we have to take action; and once we take the Lord's hand, He can lead us. He can only do so much, take us so far, until we have to take an active role in our own lives and in our own fate. But, we cannot do it alone. We need help. We need help to learn the most basics of the eternal life that we strive for. It does not come naturally! Or does it?

Isaak was obviously bright. We could tell that before we could see something was wrong. What we hadn't discovered yet was that his keen intellect would be a great asset to him as he conquered a debilitating disorder. Isaak learned to read before he could talk. If we handed him a word on an index card, he would read it out loud; but he wouldn't know what it meant nor ever use it in conversation. As we discovered he could read, we decided that through this, we could also teach him to talk.

His favorite thing at that time was a drink from his "sippy" cup. Throughout the day, he'd go into the kitchen and begin to whine and cry. He would not say anything; he would not even point to what he wanted. He would just cry. If I was lucky, he might take my hand and put in on the refrigerator—using my hand as a tool. One day I wrote the word drink on an index card and waited for the opportunity. Next time he began to whine in the kitchen, I came in to him and handed him the index card. He read the word, but continued to whine. The instant he read it, though, I handed him the drink and gave him lots of praise. He got this look on his face. I could see the light go on. This word means something. I can use it to get what I want. Soon, I was labeling the house with cards. Everything was labeled from wall to door to table. As fast as I could label them, he would learn them. Next, I made index cards with various words that he would need to use during the day: sit, sing, night-night, eat, bath. Then, during the day when something was asked of him, I would flip the ring of cards to that word. He would read it and comply. Suddenly, he was obeying commands! He was sitting better during circle time and other group instruction because he knew what was being required of him! I used written schedules so he could see what activity was next. His difficulties with transitions improved.

Things went along this way for some time. I'd discover new ways to use his advanced reading skills to help him. As he progressed and his language finally began to expand, I was able to use social stories and written rules to help him understand more complex social situations. By capitalizing on his strengths, I could help his weaknesses improve. He could hand me a challenge, and I could hand him the right tools to overcome it!

I decided learning did come naturally to him because whenever he did learn something, he easily integrated the lesson. He didn't have to struggle to relearn things he had already mastered. Once he learned something, he could use it. For him, the well just hadn't been tapped. Perhaps his special well was located in a different place from that of other children. We had more work to find it and to access it. Once the water was drawn, though, it was sweet and precious.

There were plenty of naysayers—especially in those early years when Isaak showed much more autistic behavior. There were many who thought I expected too much of him, that I was setting him up for failure. There were also many persons who were quick to discount his unusual abilities by calling them "splinter skills"; or, conversely, they would not even believe that he was truly exhibiting those skills. However, I knew him best; and I was the one entitled to revelation on his behalf.

The world of autism has so much chaos; so many experts disagree on such things as symptoms, diagnosis, and treatment. My intuition and inspiration were all I had to rely on to discern the truth for my son. I needed to rely on my spiritual foundation to know what was right. He had an extra dose of uniqueness for which I was going to need special guidance. Each step of the way, I had to forge new paths.

As I followed that instinct and relied on the Lord's guidance, I did find the right paths. I could tell when I made the right decision for him. I felt it; I felt the peace. The fruits would show themselves as Isaak made new gains and advances. I knew when I made the wrong decision (which I did many times). I could feel the turmoil in my soul. I didn't feel at peace. Soon, my error in helping him would be obvious in his behavior or lack of progress; and I would have to backtrack and try a new path. As the years went by, I learned to rely more on that inner voice, and I took fewer wrong turns.

After lots of hard work, the secluded child I knew began emerging. He began talking and communicating. He began socializing and showing an interest in other people's actions and emotions. He began to put away silly rituals and replace them with typical play. He began to respond more to other children. His programs turned from sitting at a table and labeling flashcards to playing on the floor with a peer because he could finally do that. He began to learn more from the environment and less from direct teaching. He began to become a typical child. He is merely becoming what I already knew, deep down, he was. He is living up to his full potential.

Our blinders are on here on earth. We cannot remember life before this experience. We cannot see the life on the other side now. We can only rely on the faith and knowledge that we gain here to know that the life beyond the grave is real—not only to believe in an eternal life, but to live this life in a manner to attain it. We have to trust in One who has that knowledge and the experience. We have to put our hand in His, knowing that the work will be hard and that we will have to fight against our very selves in order to succeed. Yet, there will be successes. There will be victories. And we will feel when He is pleased and when we are on the right path.

I have come to realize that Isaak is in the Lord's hands. There were dark hours when I felt incapable of parenting this child. I had to remind myself of the eternal scope of things. He is not truly my child, but is merely "on loan" to me. The Lord will take care of him. Blessings were given to me and to Isaak in which I understood that he was sent here for a very special purpose, one that I cannot see nor comprehend. Only when I would submit to that fact and leave my feelings of inadequacy behind, could I be helpful to my son. My husband finally helped me realize that I couldn't muddle things up. I didn't have that power. Whatever the Lord had in store for my son would come to pass, whether I was part of the process or not. With that understanding, I did all that I could to create possibilities for him. I just wanted him to be all that he could be, whatever the Lord decided that was.

I recently asked my husband what he would consider the biggest lesson he has learned in parenting this special child. His response was "that service should not be based on your own agenda of what you think is right; you should let the Lord decide and be willing to do it His way. Don't rely on your own arm to 'make it happen,' but accept also that He works through other people as well."

After years of incredibly hard work and with the guidance of a loving Heavenly Father, Isaak has made remarkable gains. He is 5 ½ now and fully mainstreamed in a first-grade classroom with minimal assistance. He is not only socially aware, but he can name his friends. His language is still pedantic and stilted at times, but he can get by better than I expected. He is still unusual and has to fight his natural, autistic tendencies; but he is making great progress. The future is still not clear, but I have faith. I see him getting baptized, getting the priesthood, going on a mission, and eventually finding a righteous girl to take to the temple. I see him understanding the gospel on a different level from what I do. I see him finding a profession that will cultivate his unique learning style and intellect. I see him doing "good" in the world on a large scale. Perhaps they're just the hopes of an overzealous mother. I've been called worse than that. But for now, I do hope. I do believe in him. And I do believe that he is in the Lord's hands, that He has a special purpose for this special child and for all special children.

Not every child with autism will make the rapid progress that Isaak has, but I don't see his progress as the success. The greatest lessons and the greatest success I have seen has been in forging the path—in learning to listen to the Lord, trying to become an instrument in His hands, and letting Him do what He will with my child.

He's sitting next to me on the couch now, reading a book. He's not even six yet. He thinks he's big, but he's still my baby. He turns to me. "Can I tell you a secret?"

"Sure."

He climbs up to me and moves my hair out of the way to whisper in my ear, "I love you." He pats me on the head before he jumps down and runs off.

He may never know how much that means to me.

Elder Boyd K. Packer said, "You parents and you families whose lives must be reordered because of a handicapped one, whose resources and time must be devoted to them, are special heroes. You are manifesting the works of God with every thought, with every gesture of tenderness and care you extend to the handicapped loved one. Never mind the tears nor the hours of regret and discouragement; never mind the times when you feel you cannot stand another day of what is required. You are living the principles of the gospel of Jesus Christ in exceptional purity. And you perfect yourselves in the process."

Chapter Seven

Beth, age 6
by Meg Stout

Meg Stout is a physicist and program manager for the Navy involved in research and development of anti-submarine warfare systems. One of Meg's hobbies is family history. In conjunction with researching a book on her female ancestors, Meg has identified autistic traits in the four generations preceeing her daughter. Meg is married to Bryan Stout, an expert on artificial intelligence as applied to computer games. Meg and Bryan are the parents of three daughters.

The Gardener

By Pat Chiu

If you were a gardener, your child a seed,

Your task it would be to nurture and weed

'way wild things that threaten destruction and strife

and prepare the young plant for the rigors of life.

But a daisy's a daisy, a rose is a rose,

And the plant must be true to its form as it grows.

True to the form from the Maker sent

And not to the will of the gardener bent.

Discovery

It was a miracle that Arthur was ever born! But despite the best medical care, he died of a heart defect when eight days old. It's important to know that, to understand why I noticed Beth's vagueness as an infant.

We were impatient to have another child after Arthur left us. I remember thinking he had "punched out early" to make way for another child to come to our family; and I had plans to start trying as soon as possible. The doctor told me all kinds of horror stories that persuaded me to wait for six months after the C-section to try again, and I became pregnant the first month we tried. Because of the earlier heart defect, we did a full battery of non-invasive tests. When the baby was six weeks, I saw a tiny bean-like being actively moving around. By six months into my pregnancy, we knew she was a girl with a perfectly-formed heart. We started calling her by the female name we had selected over a year before– Margaret Elizabeth Stout, or Beth for short.

Beth was born without complication on a clear, snowy morning in March. I was discharged less than 24 hours later. At home I remember the haze of mild psychosis induced by labor and sleep deprivation. Beth looked exactly like her brother – except she was a girl and she wasn't full of tubes. And she had a calm and distant look in her eyes. At the time, I loved that look. When she looked at me with that unconcerned look, I knew in my soul that she wasn't my dead son. I knew that I wasn't in another dream of my son alive, only to have the dream snatched from me upon waking.

The next few months were a haze of moving, having my gall bladder removed, returning to work and working with the children at church. My mother, herself having borne ten children, cared for Beth during the days. I vaguely recall when Beth was around six months my mother commented that Beth seemed slightly delayed. We worked with Beth, moving her limbs in a crawling motion for several minutes each day – a treatment that had helped a girl in the ward with Rett's Syndrome. For the most part, however, we just enjoyed our perfect and beautiful daughter.

When Beth was about two years old, I was sitting in the nursery and noticed another girl who was two months older. She was busily toddling around; and when the child's parents came in, she started talking, saying please and thank you. I became really aware for the first time that Beth didn't have any language yet. In the weeks that followed, I realized she was, in fact, delayed. But she sang songs verbatim, and I didn't see any cause for concern—quite.

My own brother had talked late, and so we read Thomas Sowell's book, The Late Talking Child. There was a theory that some late talkers were in fact brilliant, that their minds were so busy developing that they started talking a little late. Both my husband Bryan and I had scored in the 99th percentile on our college boards; we were both musical and trained in math and physics. Perhaps our little darling was simply too brilliant to prattle like other children.

By this time I was pregnant again. As summer approached, I became concerned that my husband was simply not providing a sufficiently enriching environment for Beth during the days while I worked. He was at home, writing a book. I decided I would rectify the situation while I was home on maternity leave. I would come to the rescue, and Beth would blossom under my attentions. Then I would reveal my concerns to Bryan, and he would see the error of his earlier ways. All would be well.

Anne was born, and again I was thrown into the mild disorientation. This time there was no calm set of eyes to dissuade me from seeing my son each time I looked at my baby girl. Anne resembled Arthur until she was ten months old. Between nursing and sleeping, I threw myself into the education of Beth. I worked with her consistently, but after she would say the few words she had mastered, she completely lost interest. She preferred to play with her toys, lining them up in precise lines, gloating over them. She would laugh and flap her hands excitedly on either side of her face. She ignored me when I tried to "make" her learn. I realized that I could not force Beth to progress faster by simply paying more attention. Bryan didn't learn I had ever blamed Beth's delays on him until years later.

That fall, we decided to participate in the stake musical. My mother kindly agreed to help with costumes and to watch the little girls during the Saturday practices. About a month into practice, Mom said, "You know, Beth seems like she could be borderline autistic." We immediately set up a consultation with our pediatrician. The pediatrician worked with Beth for only a minute and declared she was perfectly normal. But she did refer us to the county ChildFind office. ChildFind would assess Beth, she explained. If ChildFind observed any significant developmental delays, Beth could receive services from the county to help reverse those delays.

The ladies who evaluated Beth were all very kind. There was stacking of blocks, drawing of lines, attempts to have her play with dolls, matching of colors, attempts at conversation. When they called us in to hear their results, they all commented that Beth was a lovely and delightful child. Her ability to communicate, however, was at the 10-12 month level (Beth was almost 3 years old at this point). The language she did exhibit was "echolalic," appearing to be learned by rote rather than in the more normal manner. The team at ChildFind recommended we enroll Beth in the special needs county pre-school, preferably five days a week, the maximum possible. Christmas break was approaching, and the paperwork would take a while to wend its way through the system. Beth probably wouldn't get enrolled for another couple of months. ChildFind would not label Beth as autistic, preferring to defer such specific labels at such an early age. Instead they gave the diagnosis as "Pervasive Developmental Delay, Not Otherwise Specified" or PDD-NOS.

That Christmas season was a dark time. Not only did we have to adjust to Beth's classification as truly delayed, but Beth also suddenly started to regress. She would panic in crowds. She lost what little language she had. She began to make ugly faces, making her look more like a frightened animal than a little girl. I remember being at a stake workshop for families, crying as I talked about my little girl and my sense of loss. I had read what the future might hold: feces smeared on walls, individuals unable to talk, and use of simple drawings to communicate, if at all. I was afraid. I could feel Beth slipping away from me.

Signs and Teletubbies

When Beth had been a baby, a young man who was deaf was in Primary. Since I was one of those in charge of the children at church, I threw myself into learning "sign language." We were lucky enough to have two certified ASL interpreters in the ward, so I never had to do more than say 'Hi!' and spell stuff. But I learned a fair amount as we taught the entire Primary signs for the songs, and as I watched the interpreters sign.

Beth had always been surrounded by books, and I often read to her in the evenings. After her delays were identified formally, I would read to her and ask to point out items on the page. If she wouldn't point, I would take her finger and point to the page, praising her in that high maternal voice I used to despise. I also learned to sign her favorite stories.

Teletubbies were all the rage at the time, and Beth had stuffed versions of each character. She could repeat the song: "Tinky Winky, Dipsy, Laa Laa, Po. Teletubbies, Teletubbies, Say Hello!" But she didn't connect a particular name with a particular doll. I would hold the dolls up in order and praise her as she got the names "right." But when I'd present them out of order, she'd just parrot the words to the song. Then one day, I held up the Dipsy doll first. (I knew she particularly liked Dipsy.) She started to say "Tink"… then paused a long time. Her face cleared, and she stated "Dipsy." That was the first time after her diagnosis that I remember her properly identifying an object by name.

Beth loved cookies, and it was so easy to know what she wanted when she grunted in the direction of the cookie jar. But I started to use the sign for cookie, and soon would pretend not to understand what she wanted unless she either signed or said "cookie." With "cookie" mastered, we moved to "want cookie." Somewhere she picked up that "please" helped her get what she wanted, so she would use it twice: "Please, PLEASE!" Some days she tried to get away with simply grunting, but I would prompt her with sign language to say the words required for me to give her the cookie.

Beth's words began to come back when she started school, and I would keep her occupied in church by drawing simple pictures. If she could name them, I would write down exactly what she said. Otherwise, I would tell her what the picture was and write the name. One Sunday I ran out of ideas after a couple of columns of pictures, and I drew a letter of the alphabet. To my surprise, she correctly named the letter! I went through several other letters and digits, and she knew most of them. At the next home visit with Beth's pre-school teacher, I thanked her for teaching Beth her alphabet and numbers. Miss Heather looked at me funny and said they hadn't taught the kids letters and numbers. I suppose I should give the credit to all those PBS shows! We certainly had not taught her the alphabet; we had merely honed knowledge she had already obtained.

After Beth had a year of preschool, I realized that she never called anyone by name. Cookies and other food products were now "held hostage" until she would say Mother or Father before stating her desire. We again would prompt her using sign language—to avoid her echolalic repetition of the entire phrase (e.g., "Say-Mommy-I-want-a-cookie-please, PLEASE!").

The sign language had an additional benefit – she had to look at us to see why we were refusing to give her what she wanted. The next casualty in the food wars was "Please, PLEASE!" The poor girl would sometimes have to try the phrase dozens of times before the "I, may, please, Mother," and other words were all present in the proper number and in the right order. When she became capable of getting into the food herself, we bought locks for the refrigerator and kitchen.

As soon as she learned to open doors, we had another worry – night terrors. She still couldn't talk about things; she could only express near and present desires. She couldn't tell us why she was waking up in a panic in the middle of the night. I "took a leap" and guessed that she was panicked about someone getting in her door at night, now that she understood that the door could be opened. We bought locks for her doorknob. When she learned to break the lock off, we arranged a positive lock on the outside of the door. Once she couldn't open her own door at night, the terrors stopped.

At night we would ask the girls to pray, and again I would use sign language. I figured limiting the prayers to words I could sign kept them at about the right level for my minimally-communicative daughter. I knew "Heavenly Father," "thank," "today," "family," "help," "sleep," "name," "Jesus Christ," and "amen." I would make a sign, and Beth would say the phrase that went with the sign. I went to the lady who interpreted to ask for additional signs – "obey," "healthy," "strong," "good"—and the prayers got longer.

We talked with the school about using sign language, but they demurred. ASL [American Sign Language] was not universally understood, they explained. They felt it far better to go with pictures and schedules as far as classroom instruction was concerned. They thought it better for Beth to learn skills based on general tools that wouldn't make her stand apart, rather than teach her coping techniques that were even more weird. We saw their point, but continued to use ASL at home.

Though I couldn't be home during the days, Beth had the luxury of being home when she wasn't in pre-school, and home was filled with thousands of items. There were several stuffed manatees, dozens of bears, many videos covers with brunette girls on the cover – in short, lots of things she could line up that had an organizing principle. Sometimes it was fun to figure out why she thought two items were similar. Sometimes she'd organize by texture, sometimes by color. When we'd find the contents of the video cabinets arranged in a long line across the living room floor, or dozens of stuffed animals stacked across the couch, we would tell ourselves her activity was okay. But we were pretty sure when Beth started drawing on the walls that this activity was not good. We had a home visit from her preschool teacher scheduled for the next day when we found the large head drawn in permanent magic marker in the stairwell. We hoped Miss Doreen hadn't seen the mess when we escorted her inside. We sat and talked about Beth's progress and the results of a recent assessment.

"Unfortunately, Beth isn't drawing anthropomorphic figures yet – just shapes," Miss Doreen explained. Suddenly the blue head in the stairwell was a symbol of Beth's progress, and we dragged Beth's teacher over to see it. As time went on, I learned how to clean most markings from the wall, and resolved to let the rest go until some later time.

Sundays

Beth didn't like Sundays. During the school year she had five days of school and Saturday morning to mitigate the irritation of having to wear a dress and sit in a boring adult meeting. She hated the noisy children's meetings and confusing classroom settings. She hadn't minded nursery, and in Sunbeams they mostly played with clay; but now she was a CTR, and it wasn't nearly as fun.

Her teachers were wonderful though. She had a series of husband-wife teams as teachers. When a new couple would come on board, I would ask if they needed me to sit in class with her. Usually the answer was no; they had it covered. The bishopric even called a primary worker specifically to work with Beth. When Beth saw her teachers, she was happy; but she would still fight getting dressed on Sunday mornings.

At the time, my husband was first a counselor in the Elder's Quorum, then Ward Mission Leader: both "bottomless-pit" callings that can "eat you alive." I was the Teacher Development Coordinator and was supposed to revitalize and improve teaching in the congregation [Oaks, "Gospel Teaching," *Ensign*, November 1999]. Both of us were busy most Sundays, besides being the parents of little children.

Once in a while things didn't work properly, and Beth would be with me for Sunday meetings. There was more than one "Teaching the Gospel" class when I had the opportunity to demonstrate to yet another group of teachers-in-training what an autistic child can be like. But I rarely had to take Beth with me to Relief Society (the women's meeting). She would go back to her class, or we would stay in the halls.

But then came a summer with no school. Money was tight, and we simply missed the application deadline. Beth had disliked Sundays before, but now she really reacted. As I would ask her which dress she would like to wear to church, she would plead, "Beth go to school!" and try to put on pants and a school shirt. We finally found one outfit that she would tolerate, and she wore it every Sunday that summer.

The first Sunday they brought Beth to me, she was a blubbering mess. The Primary worker delivered her apologetically – they had tried to calm her, but she wanted her mother. I spent the rest of the block of meetings walking around the church parking lot with her, pointing to leaves and yellow curbs and flowers and eventually calming her down.

The second Sunday they had to bring Beth to me, I could hear her screaming from down the hall. I excused myself from the Relief Society room and gathered her in my arms. Again I spent the rest of the meeting time with Beth.

The last Sunday of that month, I had agreed to say the closing prayer in Relief Society. I was sitting on the front row when I heard Beth's cries. I hurried over to the hassled Primary counselor and led Beth back to my seat. She soon calmed down and started playing, flipping herself back across my knees. I was trying to listen to the lesson while interacting with my daughter when a good friend tapped me on the shoulder. I turned around to see her frowning face. She urgently whispered for me to take Beth out. Confused, I told her I was supposed to say the closing prayer. Immediately several people behind me said they'd cover it, while my friend huffed, "Beth's being very disruptive." Tears sprang to my eyes, and I blindly stood up. By the time I reached the door, I was sobbing. I was angry with myself, but I could not stop crying. I was outside crying when the meetings broke up, and I was still crying when choir practice let out. I even cried in the car on the way home.

I intended to call my friend later that day; but I was afraid she'd still not understand, and it would just be worse than it already was. We had been in the Primary presidency together when Beth was a baby and had spent countless hours talking and confiding and serving together. I hoped she might call me and tell me it was all right—that she hadn't meant it—but the phone didn't ring.

That Tuesday I went to Home, Family and Personal Enrichment night. My friend was seated across the room. When we broke for refreshments, I headed over; and the tears started to flow again.

"Oh, Meg!" she said. "As you were leaving Relief Society on Sunday, the other sisters were saying that Beth is autistic. Is it true?"

"Oh… Yeah." I started to laugh through the tears. "I thought you knew –Oh, good grief!" We hugged and laughed and cried.

That week I came upon a plan. The first Sunday of the new month I brought a pair of walkie-talkies. I gave one to Beth's Primary teachers, with instructions to buzz me if she started having problems. We didn't use them every week, but the walkie-talkies did allow us to prevent the extended and disruptive bawling sessions.

Cleanliness is next to Godliness...

Despite having an older child and being the oldest of ten children, I had never successfully toilet-trained anyone. Of my siblings, I only recalled one child's toileting experience – he was three, and we told him that if he peed or pooped his pants, they would burst into flames under him. He was potty-trained from that day forth!

As for my oldest daughter, I was a single, working mom taking a full-load of university classes, and diapers were convenient. When my oldest daughter was three, it appeared she was changing her own diapers. In order to get her use to the potty I sat down with her and told her I would give her 20 quarters a week, but that each diaper would cost her $0.25. After $0.50, she never used another diaper.

I hadn't worried very much about Beth's getting toilet-trained, particularly once we discovered she was developmentally delayed. Her first preschool teacher didn't see toileting as a big deal. Beth's second year of pre-school, the teacher decided to set the IEP goals by interpolating between Beth's current level and what would be required in kindergarten. Potty-training figured heavily in this set of goals. We were constantly made aware of techniques and books that could help. We read potty-training stories and sat her on the toilet, but to no avail. She simply wouldn't do it.

The last year of pre-school Beth was clearly behind in potty-training. As we began preparing Beth for the transition to kindergarten, we realized that potty-training (or the lack thereof) would determine her placement.

They sent home pictures for the bathroom walls, showing the proper sequence for toileting. Little stick figures with soiled and wet pants were shown with frowning faces. Beth's schoolteachers created a toilet book specifically for Beth. Beth would have me read the book over and over, but still she would not go.

I had bought little step stools and training covers for all the bathrooms. We had a training toilet in the hallway near the TV room and another in the kitchen. I had Beth sit on the toilet after meals and before baths and bedtime. When I would see the telltale look on her face, I would rush her to the bathroom in hopes of getting her over the toilet before it was too late. But with all the effort, we made no progress.

The kindergarten placement meeting occurred, and Beth was still not potty-trained. After we visited the autism-specific program, however, we didn't feel right about putting Beth in it. The local school relented on their previous stance regarding toileting, and Beth started kindergarten in the local school's non-categorical, special needs program.

The winter of that first kindergarten year I tried putting Beth in panties on Saturdays. The first Saturday, she wore the panties all morning. I repeatedly asked if she needed to go to the bathroom and sat her on the toilet, but nothing happened. After noon, she stiltedly asked – "Mother, may I have a pull-up. Please?" She took the first no in stride, but as the hours passed she became more and more insistent, while simultaneously refusing the use the toilet. Finally, at three o'clock, I heard a loud splashing noise. She had been unable to hold it any longer. I tried for a few more weeks, until I got sick of cleaning up the peed-on carpet and decided she just wasn't ready yet.

At the end of January, Beth's teachers attended a teacher's conference and were given additional ideas about toilet-training. They sent a note home asking us to send in changes of clothes and about two dozen pairs of panties. Bryan put her in panties that morning. That was it. All week she consistently urinated in the toilet, both at school and home. (Having her stay dry at night came gradually over the subsequent months.)

I had planned a party for that Saturday not knowing Beth would have started toileting. It was a gathering at my home for a friend who was moving away. Several of her other friends, including the bishop, were there. There was good food and good company. Then, from the corner of my eye, I saw Beth near the upstairs staircase, naked below the waist. I scooted her up the stairs and came upon the bathroom scene. Beth's pants and panties were by the sink. Just in front of the toilet there was a large puddle of urine and a large turd.

I put my arms around Beth, and hugged her. She had noticed that she needed to go, she had gotten to the bathroom, and she had taken off her panties. She had only been six inches shy of sitting on the toilet! And the mess was on tile, not carpet! I happily wiped her, put her in fresh clothes, and locked the door on the mess until after the party.

That same weekend Beth was supposed to say the scripture in Primary–for all that she hadn't been potty-trained, she was a good reader. We selected Doctrine and Covenants, section 109, verse 16: "And that this house may be a house of prayer, a house of fasting, a house of faith, a house of glory and of God, even thy house."

I had made an 8"x8" card for each phrase, so she could read the words and so the other people could see an illustrative picture. And she actually read the right words during the meeting. In my journal I summarized the week's events and concluded: "All together a rather fabulous week!"

When Beth was four, my mother did a series of paintings on flight. One picture was an eagle, soaring over the desert. A second showed a hummingbird amidst the hollyhocks. The only painting with a human subject shows Beth, in mid-air over the trampoline, her hair in a golden halo about her head – my little angel.

Chapter Eight

In the World, but Not of the World – Jake's Story
Jake, age 6
By Janae van De Kerk

Janae and her family currently live in Arizona. Janae is pursuing a teaching certificate in special education. Jake continues to progress. His speech is improving and he now shows imaginative play. Jake does well academically, with special strengths in math and spelling.

When Jake was born, my dad said, "If all babies were like Jake, the earth would really be overpopulated." And it was true. Jake was the perfect baby. He wasn't fussy and didn't cry much. He loved to be held. He was a very contented baby. Best of all, I thought, Jake would sleep. There was only one minor problem: he had a difficult time learning to nurse. I didn't worry because his older sister, Rachel, had experienced a similar problem when she was a newborn. After we took a couple of nursing classes, Jake was nursing fine. He was back to being the "perfect baby."

In contrast to his sister, Jake was a quiet baby. Rachel had been colicky. All the pictures we have of her up to three months old show a screaming baby. She never slept, and she needed to be held constantly. Jake rarely cried except when he was hungry or wanted to be picked up. He would sleep for hours at a time. And when Jake was awake, he'd gaze at the world with a solemn expression. I joked about his being the strong, silent type.

Jake met most of his milestones on time. He was rolling over by three months, crawling around six months, climbing not long after that, and then walking at eleven months. He loved to be held, played quietly by himself, and ate without a problem. The only thing he didn't do was talk. He babbled and cooed, but never said mama or dada, or anything else.

His not talking didn't bother me. Rachel was a chatterbox. She never stopped talking. I dreaded the day when Jake would start talking also. That I'd have two chatterboxes going constantly, I knew, would drive me crazy; I thought I would never have a quiet moment to myself again. So I avoided the issue, hoping, I guess, that it would just go away. I also managed successfully to delude myself into not listening to my husband's concerns about Jake. Early on, he felt that something was different about Jake; but I kept denying the possibility. I would stress the few words I thought Jake had (even though he was not using any of them at present). One day a friend, who used to be a nurse, babysat him. Jake ignored all her attempts to engage his attention. Jake ignored her. He did not respond to his name. My friend suggested that Jake might have a hearing problem.

And thus it all started.

First we made an appointment with the pediatrician to voice our concerns. Jake was almost two. The doctor agreed that he should be talking more, so we scheduled a hearing test. Jake was not cooperative—not at all. He finally settled down with me in the little soundproof room. Little beeps and buzzes came from various corners. Jake was supposed to look towards the sounds. He didn't. They tried words next. Jake did respond to them. When we came out of the booth, the tech said to me, "Well, he has selective hearing."

"Yeah," I said, "It's the 'y' chromosome." We both laughed. Another hearing test was scheduled.

The second test wasn't any better than the first. Different, yes; better, no. This time, they decided to measure the brain's response to sounds. This involved keeping Jake very still and very quiet while he was hooked up to some type of computer. We managed, but it was a struggle.

The test came back fine. Around this time, we switched pediatricians. I liked the old one, but there was one closer to where we lived. I thought a twenty-minute drive would be better than a thirty-minute one. Looking back at the situation now, I know we should have stayed with the first pediatrician.

When I took Jake in to the doctor's office for his two year "well check," I mentioned my husband's concerns about Jake's not talking. He had already had hearing tests, so we knew he could hear. The doctor listened to Jake jabber for a little while, then told me, "Don't worry; he has jargon. Speech will come next."

I told my husband what the doctor had said. I was still determined to believe that nothing serious was wrong with Jake. He was only a little slow in talking. My husband didn't agree with me, but he couldn't convince me otherwise. Despite the pediatrician's words, Jake did not start talking. In fact, he seemed to become even quieter. His happy babbling seemed to be disappearing.

Not long after Jake turned two, my husband changed jobs. We moved into town, and I was able to change Jake's pediatrician back to the original one. Imagine my surprise, one day, when the pediatrician called. She had been reading Jake's medical record and wanted to know if Jake was talking yet. He wasn't. We made an appointment with her.

From this appointment, we received a tentative diagnosis of PDD-NOS and a referral for a speech evaluation. Jake failed the speech evaluation and started speech therapy. The speech therapist recommended Occupational Therapy evaluation, which Jake also failed. He started OT a few months later.

Around this time, we were having problems with Jake in church. He was all but uncontrollable during Sacrament meeting. He wouldn't sit. He wouldn't color or play quietly. Instead, Jake climbed. Jake climbed all over me. He tried to climb over the pews. He tried crawling under the pews. He'd kick his feet over the back of the pew in front of us and kick the people there. At times when I held Jake, I'd be bent over backwards over the back of the pew as Jake tried to wiggle away. One sister leaned over to me one day and said, "You must be so strong."

One Sunday, the struggles all proved too much. The person in front of us lost his temper. I lost mine; then my husband joined in. The bishop talked to my husband later to see what the problem was. The bishop was the first person to suggest that Jake be evaluated for autism. He also suggested a parenting class since we felt that we were losing control as parents.

During this time, Jake was also having problems in nursery (a biting problem). Ironically, Jake's favorite person to bite was the bishop's son. The nursery leader told me that parents were complaining—although no one complained to me directly. A brother was called to help with Jake in the nursery. He was to be Jake's shadow, which worked well most of the time. One Sunday, however, I dropped Jake off in the nursery before this brother got there. I was the primary secretary at the time, and I was in a hurry to get the rolls out. The nursery leader told me, when I went to pick Jake up afterwards that I was not to leave Jake in the nursery without the brother who was his shadow. I went home and cried.

I did a lot of crying that year over Jake and church. I would look in on Jake in the nursery and see how different he was from the other kids and I would cry. I felt that people were thinking that we were lousy parents, though no one ever said that; and one sister even told me once that she enjoyed watching Jake's antics in church. We took the parenting class, only to find out that we already did most of the things they suggested, but they didn't work for us. Something was seriously wrong—even I couldn't deny it any longer.

One day, I called the pediatrician, in tears, asking for help—not for Jake, but for our daughter Rachel who was five at the time. While her behavior wasn't as bad as her brother's, she was having her own problems. Every Sunday during primary, Rachel would be pulled out for being disruptive. She would sit in the hall with the primary president until she calmed down and could go back in. This happened several times each Sunday.

1998 was a year I'd like to forget. Everything was going wrong. Everything seemed to be falling apart. My husband and I were fighting with each other and with the kids. The kids were out of control. Nothing in the form of discipline worked with either of them. Then it happened! After that call to the pediatrician, Rachel was diagnosed with ADD. Luckily for all of us, medication helped her. A few months later, I was diagnosed with major depression. Once again, luckily, medication helped. And then, just one week before Christmas of that year, we received the official diagnosis for Jake: autism.

In a way, though, it was a relief to get the diagnosis. We knew then that we were not lousy parents but that our child had different needs from the others. It also caused a sense of isolation. Although most of my friends had some vague concept of ADD and depression, they had no idea about autism.

In our ward at the time, I had several friends with children around Jake's age. Although they were supportive, they couldn't understand what life was like with Jake. I would look at their children and wonder "why me?" or I'd see the bishop's numerous offspring and wonder "why not them?" How could they have perfectly normal (so it seemed to me) children and not me? Why Jake? Why did my son have autism? Why not someone else?

I'd hear parents talk about the things their children were doing: getting baptized, serving a mission, going to the temple and being married, all the things that are so important to an LDS family. I couldn't even get Jake to potty-train. I felt left out. My family wasn't the perfect family that's always shown in church pictures and films. My family couldn't kneel in family prayer without me holding Jake in what basically amounted to a headlock. My family couldn't sit reverently in Sacrament Meeting. One of us was always going over or under the pew after Jake as he thrashed and twisted around trying to escape. One Sunday when we weren't quick enough to grab Jake, he leaned over the back of the pew and lifted up the skirt of the teenager sitting behind us.

When Jake was four, we moved again. We had a whole new ward to break in! Jake, of course, came up with new behaviors for a new setting. Where he once would go into primary with no problem, he refused to go into the room—even with me. We sat in the hall for several months, watching sharing time and singing time through the open door. Jake also decided that Sacrament Meeting would be the perfect place to practice his counting and ABC's; especially during the sacrament when it was quiet enough that he could hear himself. Of course, so could everyone else. After almost two years of trying to get Jake to talk, I didn't have the heart now to tell him to be quiet.

Luckily, the new ward was very tolerant and supportive. Not all understood what life was like for us, but they all tried to help. I never heard one negative word about Jake's behavior while we were there. The primary, especially, worked very hard with him. I would sit in with Jake to help him, but he was always included in everything. The first year in the ward, the primary president asked me if Jake could participate in the annual primary program. Now, Jake does not sing with the primary, and there was no way he was going to sit up there on the stand for the whole program. However, Jake was given a line to say near the beginning of the program; an extra chair was set up for me on the stand, and Jake and I were able to return and sit with the congregation after he said his line. He was wonderful! The second year, there was no question about it. We just followed the same plan, and Jake said his lines into the microphone.

One thing that really stands out in my mind from this ward is one primary lesson in Jake's class. The lesson was on the Resurrection and how our bodies will be perfect. Something suddenly clicked in my mind. After the Resurrection, Jake wouldn't be autistic. I had never thought of this concept before because I didn't see Jake as being among the sick and afflicted. Jake is Jake; and his having autism is just a part of him, like his having brown eyes. This knowledge led to more deep thinking about who Jake is and how he fits into Heavenly Father's plan.

It has taken several years, but I have come to terms with Jake's autism—mostly. Sometimes I still cry and have a "pity party," but then life goes on. I can honestly say that I've learned so much from Jake. Every bit of progress he makes is a miracle and is worth celebrating.

Jake is very high functioning, yet I don't know if he'll be baptized. To think about his not being baptized hurts sometimes, but now I realized that it really doesn't matter. If Jake is never considered accountable, he will be guaranteed his place in the celestial kingdom. I'm the one who must strive even harder, so we can be together. When we get there, I hope Jake gives me a hug and says, "Thanks Mom, for loving me just the way I was."

Chapter Nine

Perfectly Yourself: James's story
James, age 8
Lee Ann Layton

December 4, 2000: Journal entry

James got really agitated this evening when I told him that before he was born, he didn't live with us; he lived in heaven. He was crying, and I was holding him and laughing and crying at the same time as he tearfully explained how, after his dad and I left heaven, he missed us terribly. This finally transformed from hysterical unhappiness into extremely energetic story-telling. Here are the notes I jotted down on how James says he got here:

"When I lived in heaven and you went down, I just cried and cried; and I wanted you, and I didn't want to go to heaven school anymore. And I called you on the phone, and I said I wanted you; and I said, 'OK, bye. Guess I have to go down now; it's empty here.'

"I just escaped with my rope onto the cloud stepping stones, and I jumped down on the diving-to-the-ground heaven board; and I just floated down with my parachute, and I said, 'Hm, that was just too frustrating. I was just too sad.' I landed at the temple, and I crawled in the bathroom window, and I was 12 [he knows that's how old you have to be to go to the temple], and I looked around and suddenly I heard something, and you said, 'James?' and I looked around; and I said, 'I'm not staying here.' I took off my heaven robe and just threw it up in heaven...."

James's proof for this story was that he was born completely naked!

James, who has high-functioning autism, was six when I wrote this. I treasure this account because of the things it shows me about James's soul and about his spiritual understanding: James's family is the most important thing in his life, and the temple's somehow wrapped up in keeping us all "stuck together" the way we're supposed to be. His story of his daring escape from heaven may not represent pure doctrine, but the idea that he's a spiritual "premature baby" is at least as credible to me as many other theories I've heard. James just sneaked out before he was all the way ready to come!

There is, however, one big problem with James's theory: if he thought his departure went unnoted, he was sorely mistaken. James's laborious path through this life is strewn with evidence that his Father in Heaven is watching and blessing him.

The blessings began long before James arrived. After my husband and I had been married a year, we decided it was time to have some babies; but it took three years after that before James finally joined us. It was a frustrating and discouraging time of wondering whether something was physically or spiritually wrong. Although I've never heard any official statements from the Church about fertility being linked to righteousness, some people still felt comfortable asking whether that was the cause. Every time someone would ask that question, I felt compelled to sit down and make sure I was "right" before God. But, like Job (only not so perfect) I felt right.

While we were waiting, I finished my master's degree at BYU in speech-language pathology, worked in the public schools—mostly in special units for disabled preschoolers—then took a job at a university speech-language clinic helping graduates and undergraduates in speech pathology with their first clinical experiences. At the university, I had several colleagues who were researching disorders in social language, and I frequently found myself working closely with them. These situations often involved children with disorders on the autism spectrum because of the social difficulties those children exhibit.

Nearly five years into our marriage, James finally arrived. During that time, the Brethren gave several talks about the importance of mothers' not working outside the home. I felt impressed to ask diligently whether I should quit my job to stay home full-time with my new baby. So, figuring the Brethren had already pretty much told me the answer, I studied and prayed, wrote pro-and-con lists, and thought about different possibilities. I prayed for confirmation and received a strong, peaceful feeling that I should return to part-time work.

That was an astonishing answer; so, not knowing how many more astonishing things lay before me, I decided it must be the wrong answer! This time, I asked my husband for a priesthood blessing; I was firmly exhorted to keep my job! I was told my abilities would bless many people and that because of my skills someone might be able to go on a mission who might not have been able to go otherwise. For the next several months, if I got a priesthood blessing for something else, it generally went like this: "I bless you with a speedy recovery from the stomach flu, and make sure you don't quit your job." I eventually took the hint, found a sitter, and went back to work part-time.

When James was one, he started saying single words right on schedule. I remember remarking to my social-skills colleague that he said things, but not to me—words seemed to be tools for him, not links to the people around him. When he was one, I also recorded that he had used my hand as a tool to manipulate a toy he was having trouble with. This was the insignificant beginning of my paranoia about being paranoid. Of course, I thought, I'm a first-time mother with too much professional background; these are perfectly normal baby things, and all that business about babies liking to look at your face is just less obvious than I'd thought.

James's speech and language never regressed, but they developed slowly and strangely. He put two words together at two years, nine months ("Normal" is between 18 months and two years). And, in a way I couldn't fully describe, he continued to say what he needed, while at the same time he seemed reluctant to actually talk to us.

James reacted very poorly to questions. He never asked them, and he never answered them. He liked to have us read to him; but he did not like to be asked, "What's this? What color is this?" in the way grownups in our culture do with children. When James was around two, I realized that questions were standing between us and our child, and we gave them up. We talked about what we were doing; we talked about what he was doing; we responded to whatever he said to us—but we did not ask him questions. In particular, we did not ask the kind of unimportant questions that grownups already know the answer to and typically-developing children seem to love to answer. For James, that wasn't a game; it was a dilemma and a frustration. He responded by withdrawing, getting agitated, and wandering off. When it was very important to him or to us that we know what he wanted, we sometimes could get him to fill in the blank: "James wants a…" "Cookie."

Other signs were present that I knew related to autism: difficulty with pronouns, little eye contact, delayed social development, sensitivity to noise (James would routinely attack our throats if we sang in sacrament meeting), difficulty with change. James's screaming was legendary at church. Once, I mentioned to a very nice older lady in my ward that we wouldn't be there the next week; and she blurted out, "Oh, my, it will be so quiet!" She was so embarrassed that I couldn't be offended; but that was how life was—punctuated and accompanied by a great deal of screaming about all the things James didn't understand or couldn't tolerate.

Here are my thoughts just before James turned three:

Journal entry: 2/22/97

> *James has an ear infection again. When the doctor walked in the room, he said, "Hi, there," to James. James said, "Pickup truck," because that's what he was looking at outside the window. The doctor looked at me, I translated; and James clarified, "Lookit the pickup truck." The doctor asked James how old he was, and James stole his stethoscope. James threw a fit "for the ages" about getting examined. The appointment ended with a discussion of whether James is delayed, and if so, how much and in what areas. He recommended that we get a developmental and behavioral assessment.*
>
> *So there you have it! In the nursery, James is a recognized escape artist, and they got a second baby gate just for him. The other week my neighbor who works down there explained how they instituted the policy that everyone else has to share, but James doesn't—he just gets his own trucks and plays by himself. This is because he hits, bites, and throws fits otherwise. And she keeps a truck in her pocket for snack/lesson time when his patience with adult-organized activities runs out. This is perhaps scarier than the doctor's reaction to a snapshot of James on a sick day; it means that out in the real world, James is beginning to be perceived as different and in need of special treatment. I can't really force people to treat him the same as other kids if that hasn't worked up until now. This neighbor told me she knew what to do for James in nursery because she has a friend and a sister who have autistic children, and James reminds her of them.*
>
> *So, when I sit down and ask myself is James okay?; is James not ok? My best answer is, James is wonderful. He can carry a tune and he loves music; he loves books; he's joyfully, passionately interested in what he's interested in (mostly vehicles); he's a beautiful kid; he's coordinated and very aware of his position in space; when he does figure out what you want, he's usually fairly excited to do it (he's now our official phone hanger-upper); he's cuddly and good-natured; and he's come a long way. One thing, at least, that's positive about the doctor's opinion is the outside confirmation that this is no ordinary kid I'm raising and that it's not just that I'm a bad or lazy mom. James is just not as much help as some ordinary kid.*

Several months later, I was still dithering, when my mom came to visit.

Journal entry: 7/28/97

Mom was here last week for a few days of intensive grandma-ing. Toward the end of her visit, I screwed up my courage and asked her what she honestly thinks of James—weird-wise. And she agreed that he's a strange kid. He's somewhat frustrating for a grandma, because the first thing she wants to do is sit down and read all the wonderful books she's bought him. Grandma-style: "What's that?" What color is that? etc. James hates to answer questions, and he won't do it—period. So where I've learned to work around his peculiarities, she was running headlong into them. We had a long talk about what's wrong about James that the whole world can see, but that I'm still not sure what to do about. Somehow even talking about what's wrong obscures for me what's right, and in my own mind distances me from him. But maybe that's just the grieving process kicking in, and I need to get beyond the denial. I'm way beyond second-guessing myself. I'm up to about sixth-guessing.

It took me another several months of "wait and see" before a colleague at work pointed out to me that I had lots and lots of language tests at my disposal, and I could test James myself if I wanted to.

Journal entry: 8/31/97

It's been interesting administering all these standardized tests to James. The other evening I was giving the spoken section of a language test to him, and it had him jump through hoops we usually avoid in our house—out of context questions, questions he didn't know the answer to, imitation tasks, etc. Right after we got done, it was bedtime; so I pulled out his bedtime journal, which he usually really gets into helping with, but he hardly seemed to want to talk to me at all—I got the feeling he was worried I was still looking for a "right" answer and that he was going to get it wrong. It made me glad we've backed way off the language pressure in our house.

James went to bed that night, and I tallied up scores that indicated James was significantly behind children his age in his cognitive and language development. Then I spent a long time staring at them. As a professional, I'd been trained to administer and interpret these tests, and I knew their strengths and weaknesses. I could even see how they didn't begin to tap certain weaknesses of James's, like his social difficulties, and how, when they thought they were testing grammatical development, they were really testing James's unlimited abilities to spit back things he'd just heard. I'd used these tests many times and taught students how to use them, to measure children's abilities. But it was my first experience actually sitting "across the table" from someone like myself, as a parent, receiving the news that my beautiful, precious, unique child could be reduced to a column of numbers—and the numbers didn't add up to someone "normal."

I spent the next week or so seeing James in a kind of double vision, like in those pictures where first you see a young woman; then you see an old woman in the same picture because of your perspective. I'd see Language Disorder Probable Autism Spectrum Diagnosis, then the light would shift just so, and it would be James in "All His Glory" again. By the end of the week, though, I'd had the luxury of doing my grieving in private. James, the boy of flesh and starlight, was firmly back in control of my brain and heart; and I had an evaluation date for the preschool team.

Journal entry: 9/10/97

James had his hearing test today, and he wouldn't point to any of the pictures, even though he knew them all. The audiologist said she thought he was a "keeper." So, for the moment, James's "untestability" is actually an advantage, since it will get us into special preschool. Also, today's experience clarified something I'd been confused about. Some people, like the doctor and the audiologist, take five minutes with James, and they're pretty sure he's diagnosable with something. Other people, like the sitter, say: "Oh, James keeps to himself, but he does okay. Why are you worried?" Here's the difference; if James can get away with playing and interacting strictly on his terms, he looks a little weird (looking weirder these days), but basically okay. But in any situation where someone else is in charge and he's supposed to do what they say because they said so, he goes into meltdown mode. So now I understand this, I can sort out the very many different reactions to James that I get. I can warn the Sunbeams. Also, it's clear to me now that my two tasks are to convince the first group, like the doctors and audiologist, that he can do things and he is basically a smart kid, and the second group, like the babysitter, that he does have delays and he does require special help—-without having them change camps altogether. My very preliminary sense is that down the road we'll probably end up with a learning disability or a very-high-functioning autism label.

I'm beyond the need for reassurance that I'm a good mother and not a crazy person. My patriarchal blessing has a line I've always wondered about: "You take upon yourself the responsibility of bringing into this world spirits fresh from our Father in Heaven who must be loved and taught."

I wondered whether that meant that all spirits must be loved and taught (a true statement), or that mine will especially need to be? I think I'm beginning to understand....

The preschool team had not, apparently, met a mother who pulled out her own test results. I sat down on their side of the table and appear to have received somewhat better services than some of my neighbors.

James received an autism diagnosis about a month after he started at the special preschool.

Journal entry: 1 Nov. 1997

...The psychiatrist gave me a bunch of referral sources and probed two or three times to see how I was taking it; but I really did do my grieving back in July when my mom was here and when I did all those tests. (Mostly.) Occasionally I catch myself thinking, "We have what?" The progression from "something's wrong here," to "school testing," to "school placement," to "psych testing" has been so logical, once it got started, that it seems a little too easy to have gotten to this highly improbable point. The fact that it's true doesn't negate the fact that it's way too weird! Also, I'm not the only one whose grieving should be assessed. Steve and I occasionally get embroiled in these discussions about whether special education and Social Security funding for persons with disabilities are constitutional and consistent with a free market economy, blah blah blah. Then Steve stops all of a sudden and says, "Oh, wait. I guess I just haven't dealt with this yet."

James is in third grade now and has been in the regular classroom each year since kindergarten. The school provides an aide during the morning; and he usually has psychology services, speech services, or both. He reads and spells far beyond grade level and keeps up with math. His printing was never good, but he surprised everyone this year by deciding he loves cursive and by taking great pains to write neatly and beautifully. He also harasses his mother about her terrible cursive.

Interestingly, the little boy who wouldn't ask or answer questions has turned into the boy who drives people up the wall with questions (though it took a couple of years before his mother got tired of hearing them!). Shortly after he learned to ask questions, James discovered that he could control conversations with them more easily than he could with other types of conversation. And woe be unto those who would not give him the answer he was looking for! He's gradually getting more flexible in his questioning.

The same things that bothered three-year-old James continue to be difficult: social interactions, change, noise, transitions, and caring what adults think. If he's distressed, the whole world knows about it because he screams and sometimes lashes out physically. All that screaming used to bother me, and it's still a problem because of other people's reactions; but I finally realized this year that it's also a blessing in disguise. Other children with disabilities may be quietly falling through the cracks, but not James! If his needs are not being met, he starts screaming; and he doesn't finish until he's getting appropriate services. I try to send nice gifts and help out in class. We realized this year that the beginning of every year is quite difficult—for the teacher, and for James—but by the end of the year he tends to settle in. Each of his teachers so far has emerged from the "James Experience" with a deep and good-humored appreciation for his uniqueness. I like to think that James has served as their teacher, as well.

Several of my early prophecies have come true. He does indeed have that high-functioning autism diagnosis—and we intend to keep it for as long as it helps us obtain services he needs. I also divide my interactions with his teachers between imploring them not to underestimate him and exhorting them not to overestimate him. This year, I spent the first couple of months assuring the teacher that the regular classroom was the only appropriate placement for James. The following months were spent reminding her that his "laziness" or "inattention" may represent real deficits in his comprehension and skills. I doubt I'm always right; but the teachers always know my opinion! E-mail has been a real asset for school. I can write a note at 11:00 p.m., and the teacher can answer it at 6:00 a.m.; so no one disturbs anyone else's day in the process.

I'm never sure what I've actually managed to teach James. In Sharing Time, the Primary president did an interesting and hands-on presentation about the story of the Iron Rod. The kids made their way along a rope representing the rod, until they reached a "Tree of Life." James, who at the time was immersed in The Way Things Work, was obviously paying attention and processing "at speed" to come up with this observation at the dinner table: "Mom, in a thunderstorm, the Iron Rod would conduct electricity."

On the other hand, the things that I've learned from James—or that he's trying to teach me but I haven't learned yet—are getting much clearer to me. Here are some selections.

Sense of Humor

My husband and I periodically find ourselves commanding each other, "Laugh. Laugh!" Some days, it's either that or run screaming, naked down the street!

We were at Cub Scout Pack meeting, and James was throwing a fit about something. The sister chosen to pray was pointedly waiting for the room to quiet down, and in exasperation I hissed something I shouldn't have under my breath. Big mistake! As James paused for breath, the prayer started—with James screaming "Mommy, don't say shut up! WE'RE NOT SUPPOSED TO SAY SHUT UP!" This kid is good for my parenting skills. I don't get away with a thing!

Journal entry: 26 Oct., 2000

> *We've been experimenting with a special diet for James, so we have permission from the bishop to take our own bread to sacrament meeting. We sit up front every week, and the bishop gets our bread right before we do. I thought James understood that. But before church on Sunday, when his dad brought the teachers a bag with his bread in it for the tray, James flew to pieces. "That's my sandwich! Don't give them my sandwich! They're going to break up my sandwich! AAAAAAAAAAAA!" I guess it looked like the sandwiches he takes to school. We retreated as a family into the Relief Society room to regroup;*

and after 15 minutes or so, we were finally ready (tearfully) to face the world. Well, it was fast Sunday, so they had baby blessings, etc., and they were just starting the sacrament. But we were committed at that point—part of the commitment being in my own inflexible brain, unfortunately. We marched up the aisle, quietly enough, during the sacrament hymn; but thirty seconds after we sat down, James stood up on the bench and screamed, "AAAAAA! YOU'RE BREAKING MY BREAD! DON'T BREAK THAT BREAD!" Needless to say, we beat a hasty retreat! It struck me funny at the time. I discovered a smile on my face, so I purposely left it there on our way out, though I didn't have the nerve to make eye contact with anyone (besides, they were all looking at their hymnbooks, right?).

Judgment

The Bread Story, continued

All was (eventually) well. We went back to sacrament meeting, and James went to Primary willingly enough (better, anyway, than the week before—when he informed me on his way in, "I'm going to come out screaming." That day involved the Primary secretary holding him in the back of the room while everyone else sang, "I belong to the Church of Jesus Christ," and James screamed, "I HATE the Church of Jesus Christ.")

So, Part Two of this story is in Relief Society. I stood up during testimonies and explained that the last six years have been difficult (although I love James), and I'm tired, and sometimes the whole parenting thing seems like a house of cards that someone could knock down with a breath if they felt like it—but no one ever does. My mantra has been, "I'm a good parent. I'm a great parent," but really a lot of "my" success relates more to the ward members keeping their baptismal covenants. Several sisters told me afterwards that they had no idea I felt like a house of cards, especially if I could smile all the way out of sacrament meeting today.

It's easy—when you have a child that behaves like a poster child for "what happens when people fail to control their children"—to believe that the world must be seething with judgment about your bad parenting. But here's what drew me up short one day when I thought I was offended, but I was really offending:

Journal Entry: December 3, 2001

During James's frustrated-at-not-talking-and-so-screaming-and-biting phase, this sister in the ward would always strike up conversations with me on the same subject—how annoying and poorly parented my son was and her advice on same. This was pre-diagnosis, so I couldn't say the "A"-word to chase her off, and I got so I'd sit at home obsessing on how to initiate a conversation that wouldn't devolve into that subject. It never worked, though. "Nice haircut!" turned into "Well, you know it's important to have an easy style if you're raising a child who yells so loud in sacrament meeting that no one else can hear!" and so on. Really! It got to the point where I hated to see her coming—and I'm afraid she knew it. After a period of time dealing with that situation, I overheard her talking to another sister about how hard a time that sister must be having with her difficult, noisy children. And I saw that sister run away, just like me. I finally realized that my "judgmental neighbor" had some serious social problems of her own; she had just one conversational topic for communicating with other women, and she kept using it even though it didn't work. Probably she wondered why people ran when they saw her coming. Of all the people in the ward, who was better equipped to empathize with a person like that, than me? Except I was too busy being offended! The woman has moved; the relationship stands unrepaired, so the best I can now hope for is not to be so wrapped up in thinking I'm being judged that I become the one who judges.

Margins

At an Autism Society luncheon, the speaker talked about the need for "margins." In books, the white space around the words gives our eyes the break they need to focus well on the words. In life, the unoccupied space around our scheduled activities gives us the breathing room to operate effectively—especially if the scheduled activities of life cause inordinate levels of stress and anxiety to a family member with autism. Efficiency is a handy thing, when you can get it, but it's not a "virtue," like love or patience.

Journal Entry: July 31, 1999

Everyone was in the car, and we were going to the sandwich shop, then to the park. I said, "I could just go in the shop by myself."

Steve said, "Yeah, but that would be more efficient." I said, "You're right. Let's take everybody." Our new family goal is to be as inefficient as possible, and you know what? It's really decreased the stress in the household because we almost always succeed! Why run alone to the hardware store down the road, when you could take both boys along, go to the store all the way across town, cross every conceivable railroad track between here and there, and stop for drinks at McDonald's on the way home? I tell you, if people paid money for inefficiency, we'd be millionaires!

Blessings

Looking back on James's history, I realize that the Lord has let us do whatever we've seen fit with him. We pursued diets and supplements for a while, but didn't see any noticeable changes. When we've followed the trail of blessings, though, we've found what James really needed—and for James, starting when he was a baby and the Lord told me not to quit work, those blessings have mostly come in the form of the right people with the right attitudes at the right times.

Journal entry: 13 November, 1999

I was at the mall tonight, and a girl in a Lady Foot Locker uniform flagged me down to say she's the high school aide in James's class, and she thinks James is so neat and doing so well. People have been doing that a lot lately—seeking me out to let me know that they really like James, almost as if they'd unexpectedly discovered a cleverly hidden treasure, and they want to let me know they're in on the secret. I think the "treasure" is gradually working its way out of the ground, and some of the sparkly parts are becoming visible in the right light.

On the day he started pre-school, James had a priesthood blessing in which he was promised, "You may never be perfectly like everyone else, but you will always be perfectly yourself." I don't know if "never" and "always" reflect the Lord's time, or ours; but I am comforted by the phrase "perfectly yourself"—a goal both more reasonable and more fun than "perfectly like everyone else."

Another priesthood blessing that has resonated for us was given to me, in the car, right before an educational placement meeting for James. My husband was inspired to bless me, "You may not get everything you want, but you will get everything you need." This has been true every year since then—with a good deal of work and monitoring on our part.

During the last few months of kindergarten, James's support services— the classroom aide and his psychology and speech services—were not working out the way we'd envisioned them when we wrote the educational plan. James's behavior was deteriorating, and I'd scheduled a big meeting with all the people on his team to discuss his need for more help in the classroom. As I was sitting in front of the principal's office waiting (and worrying), the phone rang, which made the principal late to the meeting. When she came in, she explained that a woman had just called to ask if there were any opportunities for her daughter to volunteer in a classroom. This daughter had previous experience working with people with autism, and she was especially interested in helping an autistic child. Of course we signed her up on the spot, and James did beautifully every day that she was there—enough beautiful days that kindergarten turned into a good-enough experience for him and for his teacher.

Journal Entry: 22 May, 2001

> *How's this for an interesting level of special education services? James's Individual Education Plan was due in March, but the resource teacher asked if we could put it off till the new second-grade teachers were hired—all three of them. So I got a call from her asking if I would please come over to the school on Monday afternoon to meet the three newly-hired teachers, because the principal couldn't decide who would be right for James. It was a nice, if inconclusive meeting—three nice, very young girls, me, and the principal. I learned a tiny bit about them. Two were brand-new graduates. One girl had had a classroom of her own—fourth graders—during an internship; no one had ever had a child with special needs in her classroom; no one knew a thing about autism. They hadn't heard the word "inclusion" or been taught anything they cared to share about the IEP process. They had not heard that special education might be usefully administered in the classroom. I also told them a bit about James, and they asked a few questions. The principal asked us all to go home and think about it. I thought it was an odd meeting to have called in the first place. My two theories are a) they're making sure*

131

*I don't sue them, or b) they love and care about James. I have more
evidence for b) than a).*

Later, the resource teacher called again to set up the IEP, and she said
the principal had chosen a teacher for James. When I asked the principal
about it, she said she'd had a good feeling about Miss Smith and that Miss
Smith had volunteered to be James's teacher. I told her I'd also had a good
hunch about Miss Smith (but it was such a hunch, based on her having
had one special ed. child in her student teaching class and wearing less
makeup than the other two, that I didn't want to say anything and mess
up James's year. Silly me.) People can say what they want about church
and state, but I believe I'm not the only one praying for my child!

These are just a few of the times that we've been compelled to exclaim
to the Lord, "Who is James, that Thou art mindful of him?" (See Psalms
8:4-5.) One of the most significant things that his life has taught us so far
is the lengths the Lord is willing to go for one anxious little boy—or, we
also wonder, is the Lord making sure this little boy changes the lives he
was sent here to touch?

Journal Entry: 27 February, 2001

*James has had the worst time with the whole "plan of salvation"
business—because you can't talk about where you've been or where
you're going without talking about the fact that sometimes, our
family is not all together. He screams and throws a fit, so for the past
year, we haven't been able to talk about the pre-mortal life, or temple
marriage, or the resurrection, or anything vaguely related. For a
couple of months, you couldn't even say the name "Heavenly Father,"
because He was the individual responsible for this horribly upsetting
plan. The diving-out-of-heaven story happened during this period.*

A couple weeks after that fit, he got really interested in death, which
meant that we heard hundreds of repetitive questions on the topic—
Mommy, when will I die? Mommy, what if I get really old? (When I
tried to dodge that one by saying "You'll be an old grandpa." he asked,
"Mommy, what if God forgets about me?") Shortly after that, the Primary
president told me that the teacher in Sharing Time had explained that we
all want to go back to Heavenly Father; and James had yelled, "Why
would we want to do that???" That afternoon was when, for whatever

reason, it all finally clicked. Out of the blue, he told me, "Mommy, we die, and we go back and live with Heavenly Father; then we get resurrected; then we all come back and live here." For the next week or two, his prayers always included that same statement, then, marvelously, the whole issue has seemed to fade in his mind. I'm quite sure that if you could see James's image of heaven, it would look like a two-tone blue, late-70's, split-entry house by the sewage treatment plant and the railroad tracks—but that extremely concrete image from his unique mind has made me re-evaluate my own view of home (though I could wish for glorified and perfected plumbing...). Heaven isn't some far-off place or future time—to James, it's exactly like home. And James is—or ought to be—right!

Chapter Ten

"Choice Spirits: Susan's Story"
Brian, 16
Cameron, 14
Dusty, 9
by Susan Jones

Susan (Budge) Jones was raised in Los Alamos, New Mexico, the youngest of four children. It is there she met her husband, Lowell Jones, whom she married shortly before graduating from BYU with a degree in Psychology. They lived briefly in Salt Lake City before moving to Colorado Springs, Colorado where they have lived since 1987. They have four children—Brian, Cameron, Dusty and Bailey. Brian, Cameron and Dusty have all been diagnosed with autism.

I first met Lowell shortly before I graduated from high school. He had just gotten off his mission and was living with his brother. We became friends over the summer, but when the fall came I headed off to BYU, and he stayed in Los Alamos. We wrote back and forth and became better friends and started dating when I got home in the spring. After we dated all summer, he moved to Orem at the same time I left to go back to BYU, so we continued to date.

I was majoring in psychology and, for some of my classes, I volunteered at the Training School in American Fork and also at some special-needs classes in Provo. Lowell had worked at the Training School at one time; and the thought briefly flitted through my mind, as we became more serious, if this was preparation for something in the future. But then it left. Of course I would never have a special-needs child!

After two years of dating, we were married in the Provo Temple in March of 1985. In the summer I graduated and then we moved to Salt Lake City. It was there, on September 16, 1986, that Brian was born.

I'm sure we weren't so different from most first-time parents. You just know your child will be smart, talented, athletic, popular, spiritual and will never give you any grief. And to varying degrees, all parents are disappointed that the child of reality isn't the child of their dreams. For us, however, that reality hit early and hard.

134

Shortly before Brian turned a year old, we moved to Colorado Springs. It was a 15-hour car trip, and I was amazed at how well Brian did. I hardly heard a peep out of him the whole trip. Of course I shouldn't have been surprised. He had always been easily entertained and played well by himself. He really didn't seem to need a lot of attention. I didn't think much of it until he turned two and still he wasn't talking. He was my first, so I didn't have anyone to compare him to. (I think I was also in a state of denial.) A lot of people had told me that they had a brother—or friend, brother's next-door neighbor, etc.—who had a child who hadn't talked until they were three and they were fine. So Brian must just be a little slow, I thought. He'd be fine.

However, the doctor wasn't so convinced when I took Brian in for his yearly check-up. "If he's not talking in a couple of months, I think we need to check things out. Give me a call."

A couple of months went by, and nothing had changed. Still in a state of denial I told myself his lack of speech was because I was busy and wasn't spending as much time with him as I should have. I'd wait until after Christmas; surely by then he'd be talking.

Christmas came and went, and we got a hearing test set up. I sat with him in the booth as they said, "Point to the balloon," or "Where's the puppy?" Brian just sat there. When we got out of the booth, the tester told me that the results showed he was totally deaf. "But I don't think he understood what you were asking him," I said. "I don't think that means he's deaf." Another test was set up where he was asleep and the actual sound going to his brain was measured. After that test we were told he had moderate hearing loss and they would contact us soon. In a way, that was a relief. To me that meant we'd get him a hearing aid and he'd be talking with the best of them. When a couple of weeks later I hadn't heard from them, I called and was told that actually he had "normal" hearing. So, back to square one!

I had talked to a friend who had told me the schools did evaluations, but I contacted them too late in the school year and had to wait until the fall. One day, during the summer, I was watching him line up his cars just right, and the idea suddenly popped into my head, "He's autistic!" I had done a paper on autism at BYU, although some of the information was outdated. But apparently some of I remembered. I grabbed one of my psychology books and looked it up. As I read through the paragraphs on autism I thought, "Yes, he does that" or, "No, he really isn't that way." I wasn't sure what to think. Looking back, I think it was the Spirit whispering to me, possibly because no one seemed to be doing anything, or maybe because I needed the preparation.

One of the things I struggled with was that many people did not believe me. A lot of people kept telling me not to worry, that he would eventually talk. But they didn't understand that it was more than that. Did they really think I would think the worst if there wasn't a reason?

That fall, as he turned three, the school evaluated Brian. I brought up the possibility of autism, but no one would confirm or deny. I brought it up to the doctor and got basically the same response, although he seemed more willing to say, "Yes, that could be it." The most frustrating thing at that time was not getting a diagnosis—any diagnosis. The closest we got was "autistic-like" or "autistic behaviors." Finally, a psychologist in the school district, who had set up a program for autistic children, tested him and gave us the diagnosis of "developmentally delayed with autistic features." When he was four, he started in the school's autism program.

Other things were going on in our lives. When Brian was a year old, before we knew anything about the autism, we started trying to have another baby. Months went by, then a year. At the same time, Lowell lost his job. It was a discouraging time. Lowell was trying to deal with his self-esteem issues in relation to being a provider, and I was dealing with mine in relation to being a mother. At this point we didn't know what was wrong with Brian, and I was sure he wasn't progressing as fast as he should because I was such a failure. I was sure that's why I wasn't getting pregnant—I had failed so miserably with Brian that Heavenly Father didn't trust me with another child. Intellectually, I knew that wasn't the case, but emotions are hard things to overlook!

Finally, as Brian turned three, things started looking up. First, we knew what was going on with him and started getting help. Second, Lowell got a job. And third, I became pregnant. In hindsight, I can see that Heavenly Father really does know what he's doing. If I had gotten pregnant when I wanted to, I would have a harder time dealing with Brian and finding answers. The timing was right, even if I didn't like it.

I must admit, I never really gave a second thought to the possibility that my second baby might also be autistic. I knew that statistically it was rare to have two autistic children in one family. Even the doctor told me not to worry.

As my pregnancy progressed, life seemed to be going relatively smoothly. That's not to say that Brian didn't have his problems. After his first year in preschool, and before being put in the school's program for autistic children, he went to summer preschool. He was aggressive—out of frustration I'm sure. On the second day of summer school I got a call from the school. Brian was being aggressive and they wanted advice on how to deal with him. I really didn't have a clue. After all, I was needing advice on how to deal with his behavior. I got off the phone with tears of discouragement (I'm sure the hormones from my pregnancy weren't helping) and got down on my knees to pray. I poured out my heart to Heavenly Father, and as I calmed down, I felt the impression to read my patriarchal blessing. My patriarchal blessing has always been important to me, and I have read it often. However, this time as I read it, a line stuck out; the line had always been there, but I guess I'd never paid much attention to it. It said, "Your Heavenly Father has choice spirits that will be sent to you..." I had to change my way of thinking and realize that Brian was a choice spirit. Perhaps he had proven himself faithful in the pre-mortal life and been "rewarded" with autism, as a protection from Satan's influence here on Earth. And another choice spirit, whom we named Cameron, was born the next day, June 20, 1990.

Of course, we watched Cameron carefully. You can't help but be a little paranoid when you've had one child who hasn't developed normally. However, he seemed to be doing better and developing faster than Brian had. Still, he wasn't quite on schedule. He walked at 15 months and didn't start to talk until he was a little over a year old. Even though he was talking, his vocabulary was built up very slowly and was very small. He didn't combine words to make sentences when he should have. But he was talking and interacting more than Brian had. He played with his toys the way most kids do. And he seemed quite smart. When he was two years old he knew all of his letters, both upper and lower case.

Brian was doing okay, considering. We were quite upset when the school district decided to discontinue the autism program. We worked with other parents to keep it going, but we couldn't accomplish anything. Inclusion was being pushed. I'm not against inclusion at all. But in Brian's case, inclusion wasn't what he needed at that point in time. He needed the intensive one-on-one behavioral training he was getting to help him learn the basics. Maybe as he got older he wouldn't have needed it, but we'll never know. The program was "reshaped" so that he stayed in the same classroom the autism program had been in, but also went to first grade.

It was also around kindergarten that I finally broke down and went to a neurologist about getting Brian on medication. I had resisted medications and tried other things first. One of the things we tried was a vitamin therapy that was in powder form. He hated it! We tried everything to get him to take it and tried hiding it in every food possible. Apparently he could tell from the smell if the vitamin was in something; and—even after we gave up giving it to him—he smelled his food first to see if it was there. He did this for years. The final straw in getting medication came one day when I was at the grocery store. I handed my check to the cashier and for the first time took a good look at my arms. They were covered in bruises from Brian pinching me. I was afraid people would think Lowell was abusing me and knew I had to do something. We found a wonderful neurologist, whom we still see, who has been wonderful in working with us in finding medications that are right. Unfortunately, when a child has autism, you have to do a lot of experimenting to find the medication that helps the most. Miracle cures don't exist.

Cameron was two when Dustin (Dusty) was born on October 20, 1992. Once again we kept an eye on our child's development. Not only was Brian autistic, but also we knew Cameron was a little bit delayed. Dusty seemed perfectly fine. He was saying his first words by the time he was 9 or 10 months old. When Lowell came home Dusty would shout out "Daddy's home!" and get a big smile. He loved "patty-cake" and "peek-a-boo". I was breathing a sigh of relief that at least Dusty seemed OK.

I breathed too soon.

On New Year's Day of 1994, Dusty had a high fever. I held him and rocked him most of the day, and I was almost to the point of calling the doctor when the fever went down. The fever went down, but Dusty was never the same. He wasn't the happy baby I had known and stopped interacting and talking. When I took him in for his 15-month check-up, the doctor saw signs of an ear infection. We got antibiotics to treat it and I hoped that would get Dusty back to normal, but as time went by, he didn't change; I knew that he, too, was autistic.

I can't begin to relate what a horrible year this was. First was dealing with Dusty's change. I couldn't believe that Heavenly Father would do this to me. I already had one child that was autistic and another with delays. Couldn't I learn what I needed to learn from just one child's having autism? (The answer to that, I see now, is no). This just wasn't fair! At least this time when I told my doctor my suspicions, he had enough faith in me to believe me. It took a few months, but I got Dusty some help and started him in a special needs playgroup, along with getting him some therapy.

The second thing was that a few months after getting Dusty going, Cameron was tested again; this time he was given the diagnosis of autism. This was just too much. I knew he was delayed in some areas, but smart— he was reading by now at only four years old. Certainly he couldn't be autistic. I thought the psychologist who tested him was just trying to make him look as bad as possible since he was getting the testing to see if he qualified for assistance. However, as I looked at him more I could see it. Of all my kids, he was the one who had the hardest time with change. When we moved into our house from an apartment he did fine until bath time, but then he refused to get into the tub. This went on for weeks. We had to lift him into the tub kicking and screaming. He was fine at preschool unless they had a program or activity where parents were invited. If he saw me there he refused to go into the classroom. I wasn't part of the routine. When he got to preschool he would run over and grab a little stop sign from a construction set and hold it the whole time he was there. One year, on Mother's Day of all days, he refused to go to Primary. He had found a blue thread during Sacrament Meeting and had lost it at some point on his way to Primary. He was so distressed he had lost his little blue thread!

And then there was his speech. Not only was he delayed in speech, but also his speech was odd. Sometimes what he said made no sense at all. He never used pronouns but would say things like "It's Cameron's" instead of "It's mine" or "Cameron wants the book" instead of "I want the book." He never said "yes." For example, if I asked him if he wanted spaghetti he'd say "spaghetti?" But if I asked him if he wanted sauce on the spaghetti, he'd say "no" if he didn't. He never conversed. He wouldn't answer questions or listen in any way to what you had to say. I wouldn't have a clue what he had done that day in school except for what the teachers told me. I can remember the day I picked him up from kindergarten and asked him (never expecting an answer) what he did and he said "apples." I knew they were doing a unit on apples, so that was a big step.

In addition to getting diagnoses of autism for Cameron and Dusty that year, I was having a very difficult time with Brian turning eight. It's just a given in the LDS church that when children turn eight they're baptized. A big deal is made out of it. However, I knew it wasn't going to be that simple with Brian. He couldn't talk, much less answer questions at a baptism interview. Testing showed him functioning around the level of a 2-year-old. Weren't children baptized at eight because they were considered accountable for their actions and could understand what they were doing? Brian couldn't.

Up to this point I had been pleased with what our ward was doing for Brian. When he had turned three and should have gone on to Sunbeams from the nursery, he was allowed to stay in the nursery. This was the most logical place for him. It was at this time that I was called to work in the nursery. This was the only time I have said no to a calling. I came up with a stupid excuse for not accepting, when I should have just told the real reason. As long as it was just Brian (Cameron wasn't born yet) I didn't see the differences between him and other children his age and it wasn't as hard to deal with his delays. When I substituted in the nursery, however, it became painfully obvious. The two times I did substitute, I came home in tears. I just couldn't do that week after week!

I've always felt a little bit guilty about not accepting that calling, and yet emotionally I was not at a point I could deal with it. When I declined, the response was something along the lines of "Well, we kind of wondered with Brian in there and all." Perhaps if they had pushed it a little more I would have accepted. I guess I'll never know. But leaders need to be sensitive about the emotions of parents who may be new to autism (or any other special need). For some it may be no problem, but for others like me, it may be more than they can deal with emotionally. That isn't to say they can't ever deal with it—it just may not be the time at that particular moment.

When Brian became too old for the nursery, the Primary called a person to work with him. We went through a lot of trial and error. Our first experience was having a person that stayed with him during all of Primary. Brian and his teacher spent all their time in one room and basically the teacher was a babysitter—not the best of situations, but at least the ward was trying. Then we moved forward a little bit by trying to get Brian into the Primary class. I went in and talked with the kids about him. Then a teacher was called who took it upon himself to really work with Brian. He took Brian to class and expected positive things from him. Eventually Brian improved enough that his teacher became the teacher for the entire class. Everyone seemed to accept his odd behaviors, and I think the children learned some important lessons. And then a terrible thing happened—the ward boundaries changed and his teacher went off to a different ward.

Up until that point the ward had worked with us. But as Brian approached his eighth birthday, no one had a word to say to us. I was the one who did the research on where the church stood on kids like this and baptism. What I found was:

"To be eligible for baptism, a child must be at least eight years of age and mentally capable of being held accountable...

Severely autistic children present a special problem. The child is not retarded in the usual sense, but his ability to communicate is so disrupted that it is often impossible to know just how much the child understands... Priesthood leaders may find it necessary to delay or deny approval when they cannot conduct a proper interview to determine worthiness and accountability.

Local priesthood authorities should seek the Spirit in deciding whether or not to approve baptism. Generally, baptism should not be administered when the individual does not understand the significance of the covenant; the ordinance would be a meaningless ritual...

If a child is mentally handicapped, not accountable, and not baptized by his ninth birthday, the record is marked "Not accountable"..." 1

Maybe leaders felt uncomfortable approaching us about it, or maybe they just didn't know themselves. It would have been nice, however, if something had been said to us. I was hurt by, and maybe oversensitive to, everyone's ignoring the fact he was turning eight. The year between the time he turned seven and eight was difficult. I watched as cousins, Primary classmates and friends' children were baptized. Such a big deal was made out of it and rightly so. But I felt like a stranger standing out in the cold looking through a window at a party around a warm fire—I was no part of it. For the first time in his life, Brian couldn't be part of something and the reality of autism and how it affected us hit me hard. At my niece's baptism I had to leave in the middle because I was in tears. I fought back tears as I played the piano for the baptisms of Brian's Primary classmates. What was a joyous occasion for everyone else was heartache for me. And in my eyes, no one cared.

Having been removed from the situation for several years, I can see that I probably overreacted. How could people possibly relate to what I was going through? They probably had no idea of the pain I felt. How could they? They didn't ask and I didn't volunteer any information. And doctrinally Brian was a little child not in need of baptism at that point. He was (and is) innocent and saved. I didn't have to worry about his straying from the gospel. But who said emotions are rational? On Brian's eighth birthday both my mother and sister called knowing that it was a hard day for me. Other than that, everyone but our family ignored his birthday. It would have been nice if someone else had noticed.

But then something happened. After the last child in his Primary class was baptized, it was like a burden was lifted. I think, after five years of knowing of his autism, I finally really accepted it. I was finally at peace, and it didn't seem to bother me anymore. And the fact that Cameron and Dusty were also autistic didn't seem to bother me as much either.

So we went on with life. Cameron started kindergarten in the regular class without an aide. I was very hesitant about this, but he had a wonderful teacher who seemed to know exactly how far to push the children and what their limitations were. Of course he had his struggles, but he did better than I ever would have dreamed. I volunteered in his classroom in kindergarten, first, and second grades and saw the progress. He never really had friends, though, and that was even a goal on his IEP. He didn't seem to be bothered by it. He started using pronouns; and when he talked, he began to make more sense. He had to keep track of the phases of the moon in kindergarten and developed a love of astronomy that persists today.

I had accepted autism, but that didn't mean I didn't have hard times— mostly in the form of Dusty. He's such a lovable kid, but he has definitely been a challenge.

Shortly after he turned three, he entered a stage where he didn't want to change clothes. It didn't matter what he had on—he didn't want out of it. We got to the point that he would often go to bed in whatever clothes he had on during the day and often went to preschool in his pajamas. This created a problem when it came to changing diapers. Even pulling his pants down created major problems! At the least sign of having his clothes changed he would start a tantrum. It would take two of us to hold him down and get the task accomplished. Afterwards I would try to calm him down and show love to him by holding him in my lap facing me. I learned that was a mistake. He would bite my shoulders! So I would turn him around, cross his arms, and put mine over his. He would bite my arms. So I'd do a kind of straightjacket hold by crossing his arms in front of him and holding his hands so that my arms were out of the way. He would bite his arms. We eventually got to the point we'd put him in his room and let him cry and scream. He'd pull out every drawer in his dresser and throw the clothes around (we eventually bolted the dresser to the wall). He'd get in the closet and throw whatever he could reach. Miraculously, he never broke a window. These tantrums happened daily for over two weeks and lasted anywhere from 45 minutes to two hours. Every few minutes I'd open the door to check on him. Either I'd be greeted with screaming and something thrown at me, in which case I'd close the door and wait, or, after enough time would pass, he'd come to get a hug and melt in my arms. He also "challenged" us by pulling down his pants, pooping on the carpet and smearing it all over.

As can be imagined, this was an extremely stressful time. We had consulted everyone we could think of for ideas, but none seemed to work. It was time to call the neurologist. I don't know how we got in so quickly. They must have heard the desperation in my voice. But shortly after we got him on some medication, the tantrums, at least of that degree, stopped.

But Dusty wasn't done yet. The summer came, and he learned to climb. And he was very quick. Literally in the time from when, looking out the kitchen window, I'd see him start to climb the fence to the time I ran outside he was over. We have a wooden fence, and he would stick his little fingers between the boards and climb up and over. He loved to go over the back fence to a railroad tie used for a retaining wall, and then jump six feet or so into the neighbor's backyard in the cul-de-sac behind us. He'd then go exploring. He'd just walk into people's houses and sit on the couch. After this happened a few times, the neighbors got our phone number and we'd often get a call ("Dusty's down here") and go and pick him up. We got to know a lot of neighbors. He'd also pick a side fence and climb over that, going into the neighbor's back yard and climbing to the next one. He'd then go through their back door and often raid their refrigerator. Of course it was shocking to them the first time it happened, but everyone seemed to have a sense of humor and they'd just bring him back. Everyone, that is, except our one neighbor. She just didn't like people in general. She was very territorial and literally couldn't stand to have anyone step on her yard. She had two rotweillers in her back yard. And Dusty loved them. Fortunately, the dogs were nicer than their owner, and they loved Dusty. It did cause me to skip a heartbeat or two the first time I looked over the fence and saw him sitting on the back of one of the dogs pulling its ear. It was also fortunate that the neighbor worked in Denver and was gone most of the day.

As can be imagined, finding a babysitter for this crew of ours was challenging. However, the youth of the ward seemed up to the challenge.

We made sure we paid well. Dusty escaped from them, but I couldn't (and didn't) get upset, since he was always escaping from me. We tried everything to keep him corralled. We put on window locks and door locks. We put up wood on the fence where there were the biggest gaps to put his fingers in. We even had an alarm on the door to let us know when it was opened. Dusty always found a way to get out.

And then he discovered he could climb the tree out onto the roof. Sometimes he'd get back down on his own, but often we'd have to get a ladder and get him down. He thought it was a great game. At Christmastime we found him sitting in the chimney. It got to the point that even the neighbors were used to it. At first they'd come running over, saying, "Do you know Dusty's on the roof?" but soon they just waved to him and said, "Hi, Dusty!" We put chicken wire over the chimney so he couldn't go down it again, and we cut some of the limbs off the tree that went right over the house, but he just climbed higher and dropped down. When he was in nursery (like Brian, he stayed an extra year) he eluded the person watching him and got out on to the roof of the stake center. We're still not entirely sure how he pulled that one off.

When Dusty was born I had always imagined we'd have another baby. Both Lowell and I had wanted at least four children. However, money was an issue at first, and then came Dusty's tantrums. After one of these I said to Lowell "There's just no way I can have another baby. I can't even handle what we've got!" It hurt to say that. I had really wanted another one. It took maybe a year to accept that decision enough to have a garage sale and get rid of the baby stuff. Even then I held onto a few things. Soon I was very happy with the decision. I felt the family was complete and began to look forward to the time all the kids would be in school all day at the same time. Dusty was in preschool at the time, and that was a much-needed break. For about a year I didn't give a second thought to having another baby.

And then the feelings came.

I had these feelings that we were supposed to have another baby. Had I gotten them a year before I would have been glad. However, at this point I was not. Over and over I pushed the thoughts away, but they persisted. Finally I could ignore them no more and mentioned my feelings to Lowell. We did what we're supposed to do—we "searched it out in our minds." We made the pros and cons lists. The con list was huge. Foremost was the fear of having another autistic child. After all, we were batting a thousand up to this point. Despite the improvements in Dusty's behaviors (no more tantrums and very little climbing), I was already feeling overwhelmed as it was, without adding a baby to the mix. There were concerns about room in our house and money. Dusty was already four years old, and I didn't want such a large gap between children. And as much as I hate to admit it, I was concerned about what people would think, especially the professionals who had advised us to not have more children. The only thing on the pro list was that I felt I was receiving promptings to have another baby.

Of course we fasted and prayed. When we met at the end of that period, we agreed that if one of us felt we shouldn't have a baby, we wouldn't. We both felt we should. I had always suspected that Lowell wanted another baby, even after I had said, "No more!" but he's a wonderful man and respected my feelings. He knew that I was the one who dealt with the autism most. He never pushed it. But now we both knew and agreed that we would give it a try, but only for one year. Deep inside, I was hoping that I would have the same difficulties getting pregnant that I had had getting pregnant with Cameron and thus wouldn't even have to deal with it. Still, I was able to tell the Lord, "Thy will be done," and I knew that whatever happened, the Lord knew I could handle it. While I know many people were sure that this prompting meant there was an autism-free child waiting to come to us, I never felt that way. I was very well aware that we could have another autistic child. However, I also knew that if we did, it was what Heavenly Father wanted for us and since he doesn't give us more than we can bear (although sometimes we think otherwise), I could handle it.

The last month we agreed to try, I got pregnant. Almost immediately I slipped into a mild depression. When I had been pregnant with Dusty I suffered a severe, although brief, bout of depression. The pregnancy hormones must affect me that way. The depression I had during this pregnancy was never severe, but it never lifted either. I could never get excited about the thoughts of holding a newborn like I had with my other children. And I'm sure the circumstances behind the decision to get pregnant weren't helping either. I had always been ambivalent about it. I was also older and suffered the negative effects of pregnancy. The responses to our announcement were pretty much what I had expected— mostly shock and disbelief. Many people seemed genuinely happy for us, but I could feel disapproval from many others.

On July 12, 1999, our only girl, Bailey, was born. With her birth the clouds of depression lifted, and I was happy to have her and loved her to pieces.

Everyone was watching her development. I don't think there's ever been a little girl who has been so scrutinized. Of course I was anxious. The doctor kept a close eye on her. She seemed okay. My anxiety probably reached its peak at about the time she turned 15 months. Up to that point she had developed normally. If anything, she was ahead in most areas, including speech. But that was also the point Dusty had his fever and went downhill. When I took her in for her check-up, it was time for her MMR shot. This was near the height of reports that the MMR shot caused autism. I have never really believed this, especially when I looked more into it, but as I said before, mothers can be totally unreasonable. Intellectually, I was 99.99% sure it had nothing to do with autism, but that .01% was enough to make me balk. Fortunately, I had an understanding doctor who said I was being perfectly reasonable under the circumstances and had no problem with that decision. She did receive the MMR when she was four without any negative effects.

Where is our family now? Brian is in high school. He still doesn't talk and I know the chances he ever will are practically zero. Signing never really worked with him, but we are currently working on the PECS system and he is doing better than anyone ever expected. We did go through a rough time when he was about 13 years old and the hormones kicked in. Imagine raging hormones in the (very large) body of a 13-year-old who has the mentality and impulse control of a 3 year old. He would rub up against people, or take their hand and try to put it on his privates. It made for some embarrassing moments. With some time, work and effort we've overcome that problem. Currently, we're working on helping him develop skills for a job when he becomes an adult. There was a time I wouldn't have thought it possible for him to have a job, but I believe it can happen now. It may be something like picking up trash, wiping tables or sorting, but at least it will be something.

I'm starting to gather information about what will be done for him as an adult. I love him dearly, but don't want to be taking care of him 24 hours a day for the rest of my life. We seemed to have found a medication that works well for him (Tegretol) and most of the time he's a calm, sweet young man, which is good since he is taller than his dad now. When I imagine him in the premortal life, I can see him loving people into the right choice.

I have had two experiences where I have seen him for who he truly is. The first was when he was maybe 9 or 10 years old. Lowell was roughhousing with the boys on the floor. Brian was right in there with the others. There was just something different about him as he played. I can't describe it, but the whole scene was a typical family scene that autism wasn't a part of. The other was his first week of high school. He got off the bus, and it was just the two of us since the other two boys were at school and Bailey was taking a nap. We headed for the kitchen (he is a teenaged boy, after all), and I turned around to say something to him. There was a look on his face I had never seen before. I could see in his eyes something different. I fully expected him to tell me about his day, just like any other teenager would. I really did. He didn't, of course. I don't know if the veil was lifted from my eyes or if there really was a change in him. Whatever happened didn't last long, but I will never forget it.

If there was ever a case for outgrowing autism, Cameron is it. He doesn't have the unusual speech patterns he did before. Even in fourth grade his conversation was a little off, but now that he's going into eighth grade you wouldn't notice anything. He's an intelligent boy and has done well in school and was even in advanced math last year. His biggest problem is his absent-mindedness. He has an incredible mind for remembering facts, but he can't remember to bring a pencil to class or to take his trumpet to trumpet lessons. His motor skills are not quite up to par. He'll never be picked first for the team. His handwriting is awful, but teachers are pretty good about letting him type assignments. In fact, when he took the state assessment in writing, he was allowed to type it instead of write it out. He does get obsessive about certain things, mostly topics he wants to talk about. Having to have the same routine doesn't seem to be a priority anymore. There were some worries that when he started middle school it would be tough on him to change classes and teachers and have a locker, but he loves the changes.

We did have problems in seventh grade. He was always forgetting to hand in assignments, even ones he did right there in class. As a result, his grades suffered. We had meetings with teachers and we contemplated trying to get an IEP for him again (his IEPs were stopped because he was doing so well). After prayer and some time at the temple, however, we went against everyone's advice and decided to not pursue that course.

Maybe if things don't go well this year we'll consider it, but I have plans to meet with his teachers and try and work things out.

The biggest issues with him are social issues. At our last staffing (when he was in sixth grade), we were told that he is delayed socially a few years, although he's progressing and taking steps in the proper order and not skipping over anything. This is encouraging. And since Cameron is physically small and looks much younger than his age, people seem to accept that delay more easily than if he looked more his age. However, between his small physical size and his social delays, he's having a hard time with teasing. For the first time last year he seemed to want friends. In the past that didn't even seem to be a desire of his. He's really struggling, and I can see how his behaviors would cause teasing (not that it makes it right). I can only hope that time will take care of some of the situation. Seventh graders aren't the nicest of people at times. Hopefully as they become more mature and stop the teasing, and as Cameron begins to catch up, things will get better.

Cameron was baptized when he was eight and ordained a deacon when he turned twelve. When he went in for his physical for scout camp, the doctor even questioned whether he should have a diagnosis of autism or even Aspergers. We have hopes that he will go to college, go on a mission, get a good job and even get married and have kids. Since I have a strong suspicion that there is a genetic cause of autism in our family, he may consider adoption over passing on the genes.

Dusty is now eleven and in fifth grade. Since Dusty's medications have caused weight gain, his climbing days are over. He still presents us with plenty of challenges. In fact, even though he is higher functioning than Brian, he's definitely been more of a challenge. He's not much on conversation since he repeats most of what he hears, but he can verbally express his wants and needs. He still wets his pants, not because he's not capable of being dry—it's just not a priority to him. He's headstrong and stubborn, and it's very difficult to get him to change. He's aggressive and often hits others, his siblings getting the brunt of it, although he's making improvements in that area. It has made for some rude comments from others, however. One day a woman said "Well, I teach my children not to hit," as if I was teaching Dusty to hit. I have never had experiences with Dusty where I truly see who Dusty is, like I did with Brian. Perhaps it would make it easier to deal with the rest. I can see him in the war in heaven though. His tactic would be to go up to someone and say something like "C'mon you idiot! You know what's right. Just get off your behind and do it!"

Not all is bad with Dusty. He definitely provides entertainment. Most of our stories are "Dusty Stories." He makes us laugh and also makes others laugh. A friend tells of the time I was taking Dusty out from sacrament meeting. He knew he was in trouble and as I went out the door he shot out his arms so I couldn't go through the door. I grabbed them and he shot out his legs. My friend tells me their whole family was laughing, even though she knows it wasn't funny for me at the time. Another time he came up to her, lifted up his shirt, took hold of his Santa Claus belly (I told you he's gained weight from the medication) and shook it. And just recently I found out that somehow he sneaked into the kitchen during stake conference and ate the visiting General Authority's pie!

Dusty hasn't been baptized. It didn't bother me with him. As I said, I felt peace after Brian turned eight. Maybe it's because we could experience the excitement of that milestone with Cameron. I had expected to feel a little down when Brian turned twelve and wasn't ordained a deacon, but I never really felt that. That's not to say that I don't feel a profound sadness as I see what the other kids his age are doing—the youth activities, driving, dating. But I've accepted it and tried to look at the positive.

Bailey is four and doing fine. We had her tested and were told there's nothing to worry about with her. She is a handful. I joke that we were sent the boys first to prepare us for her. I think she's what Dusty would be like if he were he not autistic. She too is headstrong and stubborn. It's kind of nice to have a normal experience with a child. Our ward boundaries have been changed many times, and I can remember going to the wedding reception of someone in one of our old wards. Of course we saw many people we hadn't seen in a long time. They kept asking about Bailey, and I just thought everyone knew how cute and wonderful she was and wanted to hear about her. It wasn't until half-way through that I figured out they were trying to find out if she was showing signs of autism.

She attended preschool last year and her teacher commented on how nurturing she was. Maybe it's because of her brothers. I do worry for her in later years. Already she has a friend that won't come to our house because she's afraid of Dusty. That could be a difficult thing for Bailey to deal with as she gets older. I think she'll be okay, though.

What have I learned during seventeen years of parenting? What could I tell others—the parents of an autistic child, or someone who might work with them or be friends with them?

For parents:

Develop a sense of humor. You're going to need it.

Have faith and know that the Lord is with you. It is very difficult to see how anything positive could come out of all this stressful situation. But I have seen, as time has gone by, that there has been some good. And if nothing else, I know that someday, probably not in this life, but someday, I will look back and be thankful for the experience. There was a time I was praying to have the autism taken away or to have it not be as bad as we thought. One day I was reading in the scriptures and read the following verses:

> "And I will also ease the burdens which are put upon your shoulders, that even you cannot feel them upon your backs, even while you are in bondage; and this will I do that ye may stand as witnesses for me hereafter, and that ye may know of a surety that I, the Lord God, do visit my people in their afflictions.
>
> "And now it came to pass that the burdens which were laid upon Alma and his brethren were made light; yea, the Lord did strengthen them that they could bear up their burdens with ease, and they did submit cheerfully and with patience to all the will of the Lord." (Mosiah 24:14-15)

I realized that the burden of autism wouldn't be taken away; but, that instead the Lord could strengthen me so that I would be able to bear it.

Be patient. I don't necessarily mean this in the sense of be patient with your children, although that's included. I mean more to "allow time" and realize there probably will be improvements. I read somewhere that the ages of three to five were the hardest. I believe it! For each of the boys I felt there were great improvements around the time they started kindergarten or first grade.

Give yourself time to grieve. This is, in a sense, the loss of a child. It's the loss of the child you dreamed of and the life you planned. Acceptance may come quickly, or like with me, it may take years. It took me five years, from the time we first learned of Brian's autism to shortly after his eighth birthday, to really accept the situation and be at peace with it. And you may still find yourself grieving anew as you have to let go of other milestones as your child grows.

Trust yourself. You will get lots of advice and suggestions, from your neighbors to professionals. No one thing works for everyone, and you just have to study things and trust yourself to make good decisions. I know in my case I had limited time and money and couldn't possibly try everything that I read about or that was suggested to us. I have just done the best I can. And what works for one child may not work for another. For example, when we put Brian on Risperdal his behavior got worse. Yet, Risperdal is the thing that has worked best for Dusty.

Try not to be too sensitive, and learn to be forgiving. I admit that, especially in the early years, I was easily offended. Sometimes people said things that were innocent, and my reaction was because of where I was in my acceptance. There are also people who say downright stupid and insensitive things. I don't think that most people mean to be that way—it's just they may be uncomfortable and may not know what to say. That's where forgiveness comes in.

Last, just love your child. Let's admit it now. His behaviors make him unlovable a lot of the time. There are bound to be times he embarrasses you. We went as a family to a breakfast buffet one morning. Brian was around five years old. Lowell had gone to get more food and I turned around to help Cameron. When I turned back around, I saw Brian had left the table and had gone over to the one next to us. He was eating (with his hands) food off of a woman's plate while she looked on in shock. I thought I was going to die! Autistic children need someone who will love them no matter what. They are children of God.

For those who may work with or come in contact with families who have children with autism or any other special need, including extended family, friends, and church leaders and members:

Try not to be judgmental. With all of my children I found that the ages of three to five were the hardest. Some of this was because of their behaviors, but also because of the judgments of others. I remember walking somewhere with Brian when he was four years old. Someone asked him how old he was. I answered for him since I knew we could sit there all day and he wouldn't answer. I could see what was going on in this person's mind—"Why don't you just let him answer for himself?" Because they weren't that different in their motor development from other children, and because they looked normal, people often assumed my children must be spoiled. Now that Brian's older, people can tell pretty quickly that something's not right.

Be supportive. This may start from day one when a parent suspects that there's something wrong. Often when I would tell people my fears they would tell me not to worry. I don't think parents start voicing their concerns unless there is something to back it up. Why would we want to think the worst? Denial is usually the bigger problem. Perhaps a better way to respond would be to say something like, "There may not be anything wrong, but if you're so concerned why don't you have them tested? If there is something wrong you'll know and can start getting help. If nothing's wrong then you can be less concerned." Also, although I know it's a natural reaction to brag about your kids, be sensitive of the development (or lack thereof) of an autistic child. If the mother of an autistic child excitedly tells you that her child caught a ball for the first time today, understand that this is a big step and be excited too. Whatever you do, don't say, "Little Johnny did that a long time ago."

Show support by actually doing something. Offer to babysit. As a parent of an autistic child, knowing that there is someone who is willing to watch my child is a big help. If you don't feel comfortable or are concerned about what to do if they have difficult behaviors, ask for help or advice. Admit you're uncomfortable and show willingness to learn. Even little things can help. Getting a plate at a ward dinner for them so they don't have to go through the line can even help.

Members and leaders in the church can work with parents in coming up with ways to help. If at all possible work out something to allow parents to have a break at church and also allow for a meaningful experience for the autistic child at church. If parents have to miss classes at church because they have to watch their child it's easy for them to start saying, "Why even bother?" Talk with the parents and see what might work best. Even if the situation isn't ideal or it's taking some time to ease into it, at least the parents know something's being done. There are all sorts of options. We've been through many ward boundary changes so we've had all sorts of experiences. We've had one teacher alone in a classroom the entire time basically babysitting. Another time there was a teacher who was with our child the whole time, but might spend some time in Sharing Time and some in the classroom. Couples have been called to teach the age group of one of our children so that he could be with the class as much as possible, but there was still someone to take him out if needed.

Our current ward has a special needs class. Each ward is different and has different resources available, but work as much as possible with the parents.

There are some other things the church has done for us that aren't directly related to church on Sundays. The Young Women (and later the Young Men) in one ward rotated months to spend one of their activity nights watching our kids to give us some time alone together. We benefited by having one night a month, but I also think it was good for the youth to have that experience. And since there were several of them together, I think it helped those who may have been uncomfortable alone (not to mention it's an easy service project to plan.) Also, one day I joked with the bishop's wife about how in the Church we seem to have "our" benches during sacrament meeting. I mentioned that while it's somewhat funny how territorial we are, it really does make a difference with our kids since change can upset them. She mentioned it to her husband, and now we, along with some other special needs families in the ward, have reserved seating. It's a little thing, but it shows someone cares.

When it comes to callings, be sensitive and aware. That doesn't at all mean that there are certain callings parents of autistic children can never have. Everyone needs to feel needed, and callings are important. Some times may be better than others. My being called to the nursery when Brian was in it is an example of the timing being wrong. Having something available for the children during Primary will help a lot when giving the parents a Sunday calling. For example, if there wasn't the special needs class so that both Brian and Dusty are taken care of during Primary, I couldn't teach Sunday School. I loved working with the young women. It's a time-consuming job, but it also gave me a break from the kids every Wednesday night. It's also not a calling I could have done without my husband's support.

I often think of my children and "meeting" them when we're all reunited after this life. I look forward to talking with Brian and finding out what his favorite color is. I want to talk with Dusty and find out what was going on when he was being so aggressive. I know I will probably be in awe of the people they are and will be humbled by the role I played. I think of the way people have treated them, both bad and good. And I wonder if my children will approach those people, as well as myself, and say one of two things—either, "Why couldn't you have treated me better

and tried to understand me more?" or, "Thank you for all you did for me"
I only hope it's the second one I hear.

    1 Guidebook for Parents and Guardians of Handicapped Children
(1986) 34, 43

Chapter Eleven

"Gird Up Your Loins, Fresh Courage Take"
Lydia, age 25
By Christine Taylor

"An orangutan is one of God's creatures, but you carry one of His children, my dear." With those words and a pat on the back of my hand, my kindly, fatherly obstetrician dismissed my fear that something was wrong with the child I carried. Its movements were jerky, uncoordinated, spastic, and never stopped. The baby never slept, never relaxed. I thought no human could move like that, and had nervously joked that there must be an orangutan in there.

The pregnancy, my first, was not an easy one. Plagued by severe and relentless morning sickness that left me exhausted, dehydrated, and sleep-deprived, I was unable to function until the doctor prescribed a wonder drug, Bendectin, that was the ticket to normal life. I was finally able to discontinue its use about a month before our pink and bouncing, seven-pound, four-ounce daughter joined us five days before Christmas in 1977. (Several years later, Bendectin was taken off the market under suspicion of having caused neurological birth defects.)

Labor was uneventful, though I vowed never to spend another eight hours in a delivery room (and I never did—the rest of our children were born at home). Her Apgar scores were four and five; she nursed greedily and cried with gusto. None of the nurses had ever seen a newborn kick off its umbilical clip before; they hadn't even thought it possible. They put it back on several times and watched as the angry infant flailed and jerked and twisted and kicked until she'd detached herself from the offending device. Then she would settle into mild, random twitching. Hospital rules allowed no exception, of course, so the tightest of swaddling was employed to keep the clip attached and her unrelenting screams were dismissed as newborn crankiness.

Home at last, I loosened Lydia's blanket and gently removed the clip. She stopped crying and slept. For a few minutes, our little family was a haven of new-found joy. For the next six months, it was a perdition of crying and colic. "Maybe an 'immature stomach valve,' here, this elixir will help"—it didn't. "She's doing it on purpose; make her cry it out alone"—yeah, right. "If you relax, so will she"—uh-huh. Vaccinations triggered days and days of screaming pitched so high I thought it would call dogs. Her twenty-five-hour schedule didn't help, and I was unable to force her into a twenty-four-hour day. She might sleep for fifteen whole minutes before startling awake again. I had half-psychotic visions of burying her under the back porch to stop the crying—hers and mine.

Finally, blessedly, the "colic" ended. She learned to roll over and sit up simultaneously. By eight months she was walking, and, by ten, scaling bookshelves and curtains. No one had ever seen such a tiny child do these things. At a year, she weighed twelve pounds (only years later did I learn that twenty-five is closer to normal), but no one gave it a second thought. Vaccinations continued to interrupt her active life with the same dog-calling shrieks of infancy. The pediatrician dismissed my worries with, "well, some kids just react like that," and added an antihistamine to her shots. It didn't help.

Her first real word, at about eleven months, was "hi." She gleefully greeted everyone and everything she could see, animal, vegetable, or mineral. It was her first exuberant foray into the world around her. And her last.

Church was not fun. I spent the first year and a half in the hallway and the next year and a half in the Nursery with her clinging to my neck for dear life. She finally got down off my lap just before she turned three. We were delighted to see her spinning and flapping around the nursery in such a cute little dance. She would occasionally sit near another child to play with the same blocks or pull-toys; but never interacted, cooperated, or communicated with another child.

Her first day in the three-year-old Sunbeam class was a raging success. She ran out of the classroom and into my waiting arms with the only words she could find to express her excitement: "Mommy, Mommy! I love you!" Her teacher said she was quiet and attentive and never bothered the other children. She was a big girl now.

She was always quiet in Sunday school and Primary classes. She never pushed or shoved or poked or talked to the other children, or teachers, or anyone else. She might get up and wander around the room, play with a window latch, chew on a doorknob, take off her shoes and socks, spin around in a corner, or stare woodenly off into space, but never did she disrupt the class

By age four, she was mute, non-cooperative, slept poorly, wouldn't play with other children, and jerked away from any human touch. But she was intensely interested in insects, animals, books, and TV. We had no idea what might be wrong with her, only a nagging feeling that something was not right. My mother suggested autism, but I knew that couldn't be it because autistic children were all head-banging, woodwork-chewing, sleepwalking, screaming, biting, spitting, spinning, flapping idiot savants. Not my little girl! Hyperactivity was becoming a popular diagnosis in those days, so we took her to an ADHD specialist. She didn't fit the criteria, but the doctor referred her to a developmental clinic at a nearby university for further investigation. Well, she didn't fit into any category at all, so the supervising psychiatrist declared her diagnoses to be "deliberate immaturity" and "elective mutism," and ordered play therapy. Nothing changed.

Well-meaning people decided I was nuts and offered endless advice: "Just make her." "What are you doing to make her that way?" "It's a phase." "It's really all in your head, you know." "She's just your first child; you don't really know." And my favorite: "If you'd just discipline that child!"

Lydia came down with bronchitis shortly before she turned five. The missionaries stopped by the afternoon we got back from the doctor, so I asked them to give her a blessing. It was just an ordinary, garden-variety blessing except for the phrase "you will be a teacher." 'Hmm,' I thought, 'first time I've ever heard the Lord give career advice in a blessing.'

By the time she was five, Lydia was speaking again but only to family members. She also blipped onto the school district's radar since she was still in play therapy. They did their own testing and decided to put her in special education classes for children with "Severe Behavior Handicaps." Since she didn't act out, was not violent or disruptive, always quiet and cooperative, and eventually even responded to the teacher, she was declared a spectacular success of the SBH program and released from fourth grade special education to a mainstream third grade. It took two more years of "school wars" to get her back into special education and onto an IEP (Individualized Educational Program). She was completely lost in third and fourth grades. Her fifth-grade teacher was wonderful and did her very best; but even with the help of the hard-won new IEP and my help at school every single day, Lydia was still lost in the system.

While Lydia was struggling through school, I began my own research into developmental delays and disorders. It was slow-going because libraries were my only resource in the 1980's. But I learned the lexicons of school psychologists and administrators, education and special education, state and federal law, medical terminology, child development and testing, and syndromes and disorders that seemed like potential candidates. Temporal-lobe seizures began to look likely.

I found a children's neurologist of excellent repute whom our insurance would accept, got the pediatrician's disdainful and dubious referral, and made an appointment. The appointment turned out to be with his partner, a strutting, insufferable man with a massive superiority complex who interrupted my every other word with a pontification of his own and who was clearly insulted that I, a mere mother, was wasting his time. But he carelessly slapped an electrode cap on Lydia's head anyway and ran a five-minute screening electroencephalograph. His jaw dropped as he read the results: she was having ten to fifteen seizures a minute (I'll do the math for you: that's 15,000-20,000 a day). The drug he put her on immediately eliminated the tics and jerks and squeaks and animal noises; but, with those seizures out of the way, we began to see the many "absence" seizures she was still having where her eyes would roll up or glaze over and she would be "not there" for a few seconds or a few minutes. My calls to his office went unanswered. When I finally reached him at home one evening, desperate for advice, he yelled at me for daring to call his home.

To add insult to injury, our insurance carrier denied the claim because he was not on their list of approved providers. That was it. I wrote the office explaining that I had clearly requested an appointment with the other guy and that if they wanted payment then they'd better adjust their records accordingly and resubmit the claim because I'd had enough of them.

Insurance sent us to another neurologist, a generalist in private practice. A very nice man who is, I'm sure, completely competent in general adult neurology but didn't have a clue about a twelve-year-old epileptic. He continued raising the dosage of the only drug he tried until she was a barely conscious zombie; then he shrugged, declared her incurable, and told us she'd end up in a Thorazine shuffle at some institution.

Hold it. Rewind. Time to try again.

This time, pediatrician firmly on my side, I began a six-month battle for insurance approval to go to a children's hospital neurology clinic not on their list. It was worth the effort because the doctors knew exactly what I was talking about, believed me, and knew what to do. Extensive testing confirmed the original diagnosis of seizure types and frequencies.

A drug used successfully in Europe for many years had recently been approved by the FDA and was, indeed, a miracle drug for Lydia. Her seizures dropped to one per minute or less, and for the first time in her life she actually heard complete sentences.

Ahead lay many years of medication trials, adjustments, changes, combinations, but the future looked good. Something, however, was still very wrong.

Meanwhile, "school wars" were in full swing. Epilepsy didn't help to fit her into any legally recognized special education category. Learning-disability testing yielded only a slight math deficit, which is not enough to qualify for special education. I was finally told that, since she was actually doing "better than she's able," what was my problem?

"Excuse me? She's doing better than she's able?"

"Yes, she's doing better than she's able."

"Huh?"

"Look here: these tests show her ability and those tests show her performance. Her performance exceeds her ability, see?"

"Okay. You're telling me that she's doing better than she's able. That she is achieving at a higher level than she has the ability to achieve. That she is doing better than it is possible for her to do. That both sets of tests are absolutely accurate and she is absolutely incapable of doing as well as she is doing."

"That's right. We call it 'over-achieving.'"

It was years before I understood that they were true-believers in this nonsense. I am no longer angry at them, but I do pity them.

Family life was chaotic and difficult, but not always. Sometime during her teen years, Lydia decided to become a vegetarian and would no longer eat anything that "used to have a face." This was an irresistible challenge to her thirteen-year-old brother, who drew faces on all the carrots one summer day. The rest of us were rolling in laughter, but Lydia was NOT amused.

Another summer afternoon, I got a call at work from Lydia. Crying hysterically, she shrieked that the cat was breaking the Ten Commandments by trying to murder one of the gerbils! I gently explained that since the cat doesn't go to church he doesn't know the Ten Commandments, and then I tried to get her to calm down and tell me what had happened. It seems she'd taken one of the gerbils out of its cage to play on the floor in her room, then invited the cat in to play, too. The gerbil, of course, had behaved gerbil-like and streaked under the bed, and the cat had behaved cat-like and frantically tried to dig the gerbil out from under the bed. Lydia had then grabbed a broom and chased the cat around the house trying to kill it with the broom. Every time the cat got to her room again it ran in and went after the gerbil. Finally, I got her brother to rescue the gerbil and put it back in the cage. Crisis over, broom back in closet, I hung up the phone and laughed till my sides hurt. Little did I realize that her attempt at catricide by broom was a foreshadowing of things to come.

In middle school and high school, teachers followed or ignored Lydia's IEP's as it suited them. Principals smiled but cringed whenever my husband or I walked through their doors; secretaries we'd never met recognized us on sight; people at central office answered our phone calls and greeted us by name before we had a chance to identify ourselves. We were on first-name basis with the superintendent and school board members. To a person, they all insisted that Lydia was perfectly capable of controlling her epileptic seizures as well as her odd behaviors if she merely chose to do so!

At one point we sought second-opinion testing. Much to the dismay of the district's special education supervisor, I had discovered that our state offered such services in addition to a wealth of special-ed. resources free for the asking. I never understood why that supervisor had not only hidden this resource from me, but had lied when I asked if any such thing existed and then did her best to interfere and block my access when I found them on my own. Why couldn't I just leave things alone and let her do her job? After all, she had a daughter "just like mine" and understood what we were going through! As I began to network with other mothers of handicapped children, we discovered that she always happened to have a child just like the one whose parent she was working so hard to help. I can only hope such despicable conduct is not taught in colleges of education.

The State resource people were nice enough but more interested in maintaining the appearance of neutrality between feuding parties than in getting to the heart of the matter. They determined that Lydia was mentally retarded.

"What? A kid who reads encyclopedias for fun? How do you figure that?"

"Well, on the intelligence test she didn't know the difference between a canoe and a kayak."

I guess she missed school the day they discussed canoes and kayaks.

It is due as much to the efforts of some very fine people in the Ohio Department of Education as to our own, that special education in our school district is now greatly improved. However, many teachers, upon seeing our last name on their class lists, welcomed our other children with "oh, you're one of them."

How do you fight a defiant school district to get what one child needs and avoid retaliation against the others? I don't know. How do you balance the needs of an exceptional child versus the needs of siblings? I don't know. Day by day, I guess; breath by breath sometimes; on your knees mostly.

Things became somewhat better as Lydia progressed through high school, but she became ever more isolated and distant. Sudden violent rages began to appear. Something was still very wrong and was growing more so.

Her neurologist focused exclusively on controlling the seizures and ignored all my pleas and questions as to what else was going on that a diagnosis of epilepsy just didn't fit. It never seemed odd to him that Lydia was the only patient who never once spoke to him or met his eyes, who acted as though she were alone in the room.

Lydia participated, as it were, in Primary and Young Women's classes. I asked many times for her to be retained in a class because she so clearly was unready for the next one, but she was pushed on with her age group according to the book. Most adults thought she was nice enough, but quiet and "very odd." The children, of course, were predictably cruel. Even leaders sometimes forgot about her. Her YW class took a trip to Dairy Queen one summer evening. Chattering and giggling, girls and leaders enjoyed their treats at one table while Lydia sat quietly alone at another. Perhaps an hour later, I got a phone call at home asking me to come pick her up because everyone was gone. What? Well, they'd all left. Angry as I was, I rescued her and didn't look around for the others at all. I just brought her home. Strangely, Lydia was completely unfazed at the abandonment. A few hours after that, her leader and a few of the girls came to my door, pale and shaking, asking if Lydia were there and apologizing, near tears. My anger had subsided by then, and I understood why and how it had happened, but I suspect that leader will never lose another girl in her charge. Did the girls learn anything? I doubt it.

While in her mid teens, Lydia worked for me one summer doing some general clerical work and inventory of computer equipment. I was confident in her ability to perform these functions and to understand and follow the network diagrams and establish a complete inventory. Though her motor skills and intelligence were up to the tasks, I at last saw what everybody I'd been arguing with all these years had seen: her profound inability to function and interact with her environment. Her abilities, so obvious to those close to her, are so trapped inside her head that she can barely function in the real world.

In an attempt to prepare her for future employment, Lydia's senior year at school was spent in a work-study program under the tutelage of a fine, dedicated, and caring job coach named Barbara. Fast food was too fast; her total lack of social ability made retail a disaster; office work was alright but required constant help. She finally fit in as a housekeeping aide in a nursing home with an extraordinary supervisor and fellow employees who treated her as a daughter; but the job coaching she required was still intensive and constant. It was clear she'd never make it on her own. She'd need help beyond the scope of the school.

We applied to the county board of Mental Retardation and Developmental Disabilities ("MRDD"), but were turned down because Lydia didn't fit into any of their classifications. Her job coach and I scratched our heads in amazement and appealed the decision. We both attended the appeal hearing, at which the supervising psychologist explained that he would describe his findings and conclusions. He invited us to speak up at any time. We listened quietly and could find nothing erroneous or objectionable in his narrative; we only knew that he was wrong, but not how or why.

Then, he made an off-hand comment, "It's not like we're dealing with Object Impermanence or anything." Barbara and I turned to each other wide-eyed and exclaimed in one voice: "there's a name for it!" I apologized for the outburst and explained that we'd never heard the term but understood it at once: it describes the experience of an infant for whom, once dropped out of sight, the rattle ceases to exist; or a nineteen-year-old who doesn't comb the back of her hair because she doesn't see it and so forgets it's there. "Yes, yes, go on. Why don't you tell us about your daughter in your own words?"

I described a right-eyed, left-footed child with no hand dominance, who used both hands to color or write because she couldn't cross midline until she was eight, who still walked on her toes and preferred squatting on her feet to sitting on a chair, who could relate to animals but not people, who had once been accused of lying on a personality test by a psychiatrist who didn't see that her language is so concrete that a single question worded different ways would yield different responses, who perceived herself as apart from people as though a separate species, who could not comprehend her own thoughts as separate from other's, for whom object impermanence is an everyday experience. Barbara described disastrous employment experiences and Lydia's complete inability to function in a competitive environment. We could see their jaws slacken as we continued speaking. They said they'd take our comments under advisement and get back to us. I had an official acceptance letter within a week.

Well, that opened the door to needed services, but something was still very wrong. My research had dwindled during the last few years as I relied on others' expertise, but now I dived back in with new intensity, since it looked like nobody else was going to figure it out. Autism began to look like a good candidate and answered many questions, but wasn't quite right. Nevertheless, it was a starting place. Now all I needed was somebody to believe me. A neuropsychiatrist might be able to tease out the epilepsy and see what was underneath it, but all we could find within two hundred miles was one neuropsychologist who, it turned out, was light on the neuro and heavy on the psychologist. Fortunately, we only wasted a day on him.

When Lydia turned 21, her pediatric neurologist suggested she might better be served in the adult community and gave the names of a few adult neurologists in private practice. I thanked him and consulted the local Epilepsy Foundation chapter, which immediately and strongly recommended the comprehensive epilepsy treatment center at a regional university medical center. Why did her pediatric neurologist never tell us about this center during all the years he had treated her with only marginal success?

Many months later, we had our first appointment with an epileptologist, who spent two minutes before stepping back and taking a long look at her. "Hmm, something else is going on here, did you know that?" Heart suddenly in my mouth, I exclaimed that I'd been trying to figure that out for twenty-one years and that he was the first physician ever to see what I saw! He expedited an appointment with a cognitive neurologist, who took one look at her and said "autism." As I answered the questions on his diagnostic checklist—yes, yes, yes she did, she did that too, that's right, yes, yes—the picture emerged clear as morning. By this time, I had already read extensively about both Autism and Asperger's Syndrome. Lydia falls somewhere between the two, and the doctor and I agreed that the most useful diagnosis would be Autism. I despaired of all the wasted years and all the things that could have helped her had we only known. Time and experience, however, by now had taught me not to waste time and energy feeling sorry.

Lydia was born in 1977. Sixteen years later, in 1993, Asperger's Syndrome was officially recognized and added to diagnostic manuals, before which time Autism was diagnosed only by low-functioning criteria. She was finally diagnosed in 1998.

The final diagnoses are Autism, Epilepsy, and the Schizophrenia that had developed during her late teens, but many of her behaviors are impossible to untangle and determine what may be caused by which. Autism was the key diagnosis to open the doors of disability services Lydia had always needed but that had been unavailable because we never before had words to describe her.

For the next four years, Lydia participated successfully in a productive sheltered-workshop employment environment. It could be said that she lives on her own planet. Her delusions, not amenable to talk therapy, are bizarre but harmless and even entertaining. Gospel principles, though badly scrambled in her head, are precious to her. She enjoys attending plays and concerts. She shops from catalogs and makes on-line purchases using her own bank card. Her petit mal seizures continue but at fewer than a hundred a day, which, for Lydia, is good, but she continues to have occasional grand mal convulsions despite medication. Her speech patterns are stilted and pedantic, and her clothing choices are bizarre. She cannot comprehend good hygiene or proper nutrition or other people. She will never live on her own, make friends, marry, raise a family, or do so many other things the rest of us take for granted. But she is happy, content, and living a full life as she sees it. She is blessed with four brothers and sisters who love and accept her, and she likes herself exactly as she is.

Recently, though, we have begun to lose our challenging but happy angel child to a new, dark, and violent paranoia. We don't know whether she can continue to live with us safely. We don't know what the future holds.

But we do know that Heavenly Father has saved her from the world by means of His choosing to challenge us, teach us, and bless us. I understand now the meaning of that long-ago promise, "you will be a teacher," and it comforts me. One day, we will meet our beloved Lydia on the other side –– free, whole, exalted, and glorious. Until then…

"Gird up your loins, fresh courage take,
Our God will never us forsake…
Do this and joy your hearts will swell.
All is well, all is well."

Chapter Twelve

"On the Inside, Looking Out"
My Experiences with Autism
by Richard C. Chiu

During my early childhood, I spent hundreds of hours being examined by experts in psychology, neurology, child development, socialization, and other disciplines, and was tested for almost every imaginable mental or neuro-physical disorder that these inventive professionals could imagine as a cause for my idiosyncratic behavior. When I reached adolescence, the scrutiny shifted to emotional and mental disorders rather than developmental issues, but if anything, actually increased. And in all that time, autism was never seriously considered.

There is, of course, a simple explanation. In each of those innumerable notebooks that contain some paraphrased version of the diagnostic criteria of autism - all scribbled there by some expert describing my childhood - there is another notation – My I.Q. My I.Q. has been measured many times, at many values. Sometimes as low as 130, sometimes higher, sometimes much higher. It is well understood by experts that autism is accompanied by mental retardation in about 70% of cases. I can only assume that three decades ago autism was essentially regarded as a subset of mental retardation. Because of this implicit association of autism with mental retardation, these experts were blind to the possibility that a mentally superior child might be autistic, despite the fact that mental retardation is not, in point of fact, an indication of autism.

I myself only came to the conclusion that I was autistic gradually. The first indication I noticed was in high school, during a section on psychology, brain function, and learning disabilities. Autism was discussed in the text, along with the information that autistic children—in addition to the occasional and mysterious *savant* abilities—typically displayed lesser strange abilities, like recognizing a face with equal facility whether presented upside-down or rightside-up. Next to the passage was a picture of JFK, upside-down, with a caption noting that a normal individual couldn't recognize this well-known face. I amused and surprised the class with my "autistic" ability. When I turned the book upside-down to demonstrate that the picture was indeed JFK everyone else was now able to recognize the face. But I was surprised to notice that the face, now right side-up, was not particularly recognizable to me. The picture had been cropped so as to remove the distinctive hair and jaw line. Had I not already identified it as JFK, I would have had no idea who it was. At the time I did not regard the incident as being of any particular significance. But I remembered it anyway. As time went on, I would occasionally learn some interesting fact about autism—whether in school, or from reading, or while watching PBS—and recognize this or that characteristic typical of autistic children as a behavior I had always thought unique to myself. I learned of behavior after behavior that I had in common with most autistic children. For example, autistic children "avoid" the eyes of an interlocutor. In my case, it is more accurate to state that I simply forget to look into another person's eyes unless I make a conscious effort to do so. Autistic children are seeming insensitive to minor pain. I had actually learned to "simulate" pain response early on, but would often respond to situations that caused no pain, or caused pain to someone else, or simply forget to respond entirely - particularly when surprised.

But of course, several bits of information stood in the way of the logical conclusion. For one thing, I knew why I did all the things that I did. I was often accused of avoiding the eyes of others, but I knew that I had never done this—in fact, I generally made a conscious effort to look other people in the eye. I knew that I wasn't insensitive to pain, but rather sometimes forgot to react properly. I knew that I wasn't unusually good at identifying faces upside-down, I was just poor at recognizing them right side-up. The behaviors of autistic children were a mystery to science, whereas I knew perfectly well why I did these things. That obviously meant that the correlation was just a coincidence. After all, I had never memorized a phonebook or the dates associated with every first Sunday of each month for a twenty year period. If autistic children did enough strange things, they would do some of the strange things that I did. It was as simple as that. Also, I had never encountered any description of autism as anything but a completely debilitating learning impairment. I had always been the fastest learner I ever knew, always able to understand sooner and more completely than anyone around me any concept I encountered. And I had been studied, tested, prodded, theorized over, and examined by scores of experts over the entire course of my life. Learning impairment of any sort had long since been ruled out almost definitively (when dyslexia became the big villain of learning impairments, I was tested for dyslexia—despite the fact that I read more, and better, than any of my peers). All of my problems had been traced to nearsightedness and a troubled home life. These were factors in my case, but my siblings didn't share my problems and they were all nearsighted children from a troubled home.

My sister, Meg, revealed that her daughter, Beth, was autistic in 1998 . When she revealed that Beth's characteristic hand gestures were characteristic of autism, I realized that I was autistic as well. I knew that Beth was a highly intelligent, responsive child, marvelously quick to learn in novel ways. I was aware that she was late to talk, but verbal communication had never been as important to me (or indeed, as useful to me) as mechanical reasoning. I realized that I was, in fact, autistic, but immediately underrated the import of that fact. It was clear to me that my autism must be very mild, hardly noticeable in clinical terms. If my autism were a serious matter, someone else would have noticed. Autism, after all, is a seriously debilitating condition.

Meg contacted me in 2002 to see if I would be willing to write about my experiences, since she suspected I was autistic. We conversed for some time about my childhood symptoms (I don't actually remember my childhood before the age of 3 with any great detail) and I realized for the first time that - as a child - I had displayed significant signs of being profoundly autistic. After talking to Meg, I began to research autism, and discovered that - as an adult - I matched every diagnostic criteria for autism. When I showed the diagnostic checklist to my sister, she confirmed that I had displayed 10 out of 12 criteria before the age of 3. The other two criteria involved lack of interest in make-believe and social imitation. The fact that I also met these criteria was not outwardly apparent to her. As I child I would only play out make-believe roles assigned by my siblings – they could as easily co-opted the family dog to play the roles, had we had one.

Now that I had discovered that I am profoundly autistic - from a clinical rather than functional point of view – I realized that the very characteristics that I have always regarded as my best traits derive from my autism. Indeed, my entire complex of behavior, outlook, mental process, and ability is structured around my most fundamentally autistic traits. I have never been susceptible to social pressure of any kind, whether threats, unpopularity, inappropriate guilt, or anything else. This trait, the foundation of my personal integrity, my ability to always do what I thought was right whatever those around me might say or do, is fundamentally an outgrowth of profound autism. My ability to evaluate, logically and fairly, the merit of competing claims from disparate sources, independent of my personal feelings about the claimants, is no less deeply rooted in a "failure to develop peer relationships appropriate to developmental level" and "lack of social or emotional reciprocity." My ability to ignore discomfort and pain in pursuit of an objective, the fact that I don't feel depend on the approval of others when I know I'm right, the ability to concentrate intently on a specific subject long enough to truly understand it – all are characteristics that I regard as inherently desirable.

And yet, when I view them through the lens of autism, I can see how these very traits involved me, again and again, in the misunderstandings, predicaments, and outright persecutions that have pervaded my life. One of the most disturbing behaviors I had as a child was my tendency to scratch a bug bite until the the skin was raw, then persistently pick off the scabs and eat them. All sorts of theories were entertained about the large purplish scars that resulted, and even more exotic ideas were put forth once it was understood just how those scars had been created. The simple truth was that the pain of picking off a scab and the slight mess of blood simply weren't a deterrent given the ability to remove of the scab from my skin and eat it (I liked the taste...). In fact, though I no longer scratch minor bug bites bloody (unless I'm under a good deal of stress), I do still pluck off scabs. But I now wait until the skin underneath has healed enough to avoid bleeding and generally throw the scab away rather than eat it. I understand that it is important to avoid "disgusting" behavior (although I still feel no personal revulsion at the thought of licking a bloody wound), just as it is important to maintain eye contact (although I often forget to do so).

My ability to concentrate exclusively on a subject of interest led to such bizzare behaviors as staring at a dumpster (or a leaf, or a rock or a coil spring) for hours of playtime. Though this study provided me more understanding about the natural world than I obtained from classroom instruction, it would evoke hysterical reactions from those with the power to harm me in ways I didn't yet understand. Likewise—although my complete immunity to peer pressure sometimes led others to attempt to emulate me—far more often it made me an outcast, a pariah, or even a scapegoat. Worse was my immunity to authority. Teachers, parents, bullies, or other power figures could not use threats, intimidation, or any other form of coercion to persuade me to do what I did not think it good to do. Therefore I was repeatedly punished, often brutally, always unfairly, for my noncompliance (this was most especially true of child bullies, and even those who - I am given to understand - were not normally bullies).

The perception of unfairness can be disputed, but the fact remains that I spent much of my childhood being punished by those whom I had done nothing to offend.

There are elements in all this that I might have wished to avoid. Certainly I would have benefited from understanding how much disgust my habit of consuming my own blood inspired, or how irrational teachers could be about a boy intently studying the side of a rusty trash bin. But I cannot help but think that most of the unique qualities that set me apart were good things. I cannot help but notice that the most savage reactions were inspired by those qualities that I still think were the best in me. Don't we all claim that we want our children to think for themselves rather than just following the crowd? I did. That I did so—not out of some high moral principle—but simply because I lack whatever social instinct it is that motivates humans to follow the herd is a startling revelation to me. But I do not feel less inclined to value that power in myself because it is a characteristic of a rare and frankly mysterious congenital condition which normal humankind chooses to term a disorder. It is true that all the methods of persuasion normally used with a human child were useless with me, and it certainly made my mother's task of civilizing me far more difficult. I never particularly believed in God until I personally experienced Him, and I never accepted a moral principle until I understood exactly why it was a moral principle. (This was more of a problem before I solved the principles underlying "blind obedience" and "faith".) But of anyone I have ever known, I am the least susceptible to domination, coercion, flattery, or any of a host of like evils.

To my mind, it is a great mistake to think of autism as a limitation as such. In fact, it is normal humans that are "limited." Because what separates autistic children, what underlies all the symptoms, is simply the absence of the social instincts that could be seen to constrain and limit normal humans. Autistic children don't lack the ability to learn language. They lack the instinctive drive to direct all possible mental resources to the acquisition of language. Similarly, I never actively avoided looking others in the eye, but rather simply felt no overriding impulse to do so. I never lacked the ability to develop relationships with my peers. I just lacked the driving compulsion to pursue those relationships at any cost. And I always wanted to share my thoughts, my interests, my discoveries with those around me. But usually my thoughts and interests weren't interesting—or even comprehensible to—those around me.

For example, when I was about eight years old, a speaker in church gave a talk. He talked about a recent experience where he had taken apart the print head of an impact printer and found himself in a quandary as to how to put the nine nearly identical but non-interchangeable heads back into the nine unmarked holes. His son eventually informed him that there were 81 ways to put nine pins into nine holes, and so this good brother gave the printer up as a loss. He compared the experience of trying to put together an impact print head without a technical manual or expert advice to the difficulty of living a moral life without the scriptures and prophetic counsel. But I didn't really pay close attention to the rest of the talk, because I was fascinated by the obvious error of saying there were 81 ways to put nine pins into nine holes. I could easily see that there must be 81 ways to put two out of 18 pins into two holes if nine of the pins can only fit into one hole and the other nine can only fit in the other. But to put nine pins into nine holes, where every pin could fit into any hole - that was an interesting challenge! Quickly I worked out the basic principle that there must be $9 \times 8 \times 7 \times 6 \times 5 \times 4 \times 3 \times 2$ ways to fit the nine pins in the nine holes, and set about working out the resulting product. My teachers hadn't done much more than order us to memorize the multiplication table (which I hadn't done, since I regarded rote memorization of mathematical relationships counterproductive). Therefore I had to work out methods of long multiplication on the fly, in my head, while being prodded periodically by my sisters (one of whom in particular regarded it as her duty to make sure that other children sat straight and paid attention reverently). Eventually, however, I worked out that the answer was 362,880. There were 362,880 ways to put nine pins into nine holes. And this information I happily announced to my family. You can imagine what the reaction was.

Incidents like this are why I often laugh, or smile, or look intently at something for a long time, and when questioned, refuse to explain. The multiplication incident was by no means unique in my experience... but it was one of the few that I have ever been able to relate intelligibly. I sometimes thought I was misunderstood because I was a genius, but of course my siblings and parents were geniuses too, and some of them had IQs that made my own look paltry. To the psychologist or child development specialist, the beatings and other arbitrary punishments might be more interesting, but to me it was the appalling ignorance and blank incomprehension that left indelible marks.

So most of my life was lived in the mind and in the books I never tired of reading. In the course of time I have learned enough about humans, their social behaviors and instinctive responses to begin to effectively imitate normalcy, at least for limited periods of time. I can be the life of a party, if necessary, or initiate and maintain a specific conversation as required. I effectively simulate most emotional responses, and while I still take a couple of seconds too long to respond to a friendly smile, I can react well given a verbal greeting. But contemplation will always mean more to me than sociality.

In the past few years, I have decided to withdraw from a society that does so much evil that I cannot ignore. I keep to myself knowledge, insights, and talents that might make another man wealthy and powerful, and wait for the coming storm with head bowed. These may seem like an extension of the autistic behaviors of my childhood, when I would contemplate the movement of my hands as I wriggled my fingers rapidly. Yet by holding myself apart, I've developed a relationship with God, with Eternity, with transcendent truth that I could never have enjoyed in the world. Should you neurologically typical individuals pity those that have been entranced by the vast beauty and power that is to be found in the unfettered potential of the mind? Possibly you think that I fall into delusion. It is too much to ask that you let go of your humanity, the instincts bred into your genes throughout the generations of mankind, and follow me into that endless wonder. I have known that for years, long before I learned the name that divides me from you. Instincts are instincts, after all. But believe in me, in us. We are free, we are happy, we have discovered riches that we would share if it were possible. Perhaps in a better world, it will be.

Afterword

or, "Holland, Schmolland!"

Once upon a time, an author named Emily Perl Kingsley wrote a beautiful parable of what it was like to rear a child with a disability, called "Welcome to Holland." She compares having a baby to planning a fabulous trip to Italy, and then, when the baby turns out to have a disability, it is like landing in Holland, and not being able to go back to Italy. All your research, travel guides, everything is near-useless. All of your life you had dreamed of "going to Italy" (having a child) and here you are somewhere else. She talks about the need to slow down, and notice the wonders of this other place. She brings up the fact that everyone around you is going to Italy and you will always have the pain of the loss of your dream of going to Italy. In the end, she says that if you spend your time mourning that you didn't get to Italy, you won't be able to enjoy the beautiful and wonderful things about Holland. While this parable is true in many extents, it still doesn't help others understand the things that are different about autism from other disabilities.

After reading the "Welcome to Holland" story, another author, by the name of Laura Krueger Crawford, wrote a spoof on the original parable called "Holland, Scmolland!" It really highlights the differences between autism and other disabilities. Someone on one of the newsgroups shared it with me, and after I posted it to our LDS_Autism group, we began, amid much hilarity, to share our own "Scmolland moments." As they present a good picture of what it can be like to live with a child with autism, I have put them in below, after the Holland Schmolland article. Hopefully you will enjoy these and laugh with us at some of the things that tickle our funny bones about life with our precious children!

Holland Schmolland
By Laura Krueger Crawford
(article used with permission from author)

If you have a child with autism, which I do, and if you troll the Internet for information, which I have done, you will come across a certain inspirational analogy. It goes like this: Imagine that you are planning a trip to Italy. You read all the latest travel books, you consult with friends about what to pack, and you develop an elaborate itinerary for your glorious trip. The day arrives. You board the plane and settle in with your in-flight magazine, dreaming of trattorias, gondola rides and gelato. However, when the plane lands you discover, much to your surprise, you are not in Italy—you are in Holland. You are greatly dismayed at this abrupt and unexpected change in plans. You rant and rave to the travel agency, but it does no good. You are stuck. After a while, you tire of fighting and begin to look at what Holland has to offer. You notice the beautiful tulips, the kindly people in wooden shoes, the French fries and mayonnaise, and you think, "This isn't exactly what I planned, but it's not so bad. It's just different." Having a child with autism is supposed to be like this—not any worse than having a typical child—just different. When I read that, my son was almost three, completely non-verbal and was hitting me over a hundred times a day. While I appreciated the intention of the story, I couldn't help but think, "Are they kidding? We are not in some peaceful countryside dotted with windmills. We are in a country under siege—dodging bombs, trying to board overloaded helicopters, bribing officials—all the while thinking, "What happened to our beautiful life?"

That was 5 years ago. My son is now 8 and though we have come to accept that he will always have autism, we no longer feel like citizens of a battle-torn nation. With the help of countless dedicated therapists and teachers, biological interventions, and an enormously supportive family, my son has become a fun-loving, affectionate boy with many endearing qualities and skills. In the process we've created—well—our own country, with its own unique traditions and customs.

It's not a war zone, but it's still not Holland. Let's call it Schmolland.

In Schmolland, it is perfectly customary to lick walls, rub cold pieces of metal across your mouth and line up all your toys end to end. You can show affection by giving a "pointy chin." A "pointy chin" is when you act like you are going to hug someone and just when you are really close, you jam your chin into the other person's shoulder. For the person giving the "pointy chin" this feels really good, for the receiver not so much—but you get used to it. For citizens of Schmolland, it is quite normal to repeat lines from videos to express emotion. If you are sad, you can look downcast and say "Oh, Pongo." When mad or anxious, you might shout, "Snow can't stop me!" or "Duchess, kittens, come on!" Sometimes, "And now our feature presentation" says it all. In Schmolland, there's not a lot to do, so our citizens find amusement wherever they can. Bouncing on the couch for hours, methodically pulling feathers out of down pillows, and laughing hysterically in bed at 4:00am, are all traditional Schmutch pastimes.

The hard part about living in our country is dealing with people from other countries. We try to assimilate ourselves and mimic their customs, but we aren't always successful. It's perfectly understandable that an 8-year-old boy from Schmolland would steal a train from a toddler at the Thomas the Tank Engine Train Table at Barnes and Noble. But this is clearly not understandable or acceptable in other countries, and so we must drag our 8 year old out of the store kicking and screaming while all the customers look on with stark, pitying stares. But we ignore these looks and focus on the exit sign because we are a proud people. Where we live, it is not surprising when an 8-year-old boy reaches for the fleshy part of a woman's upper torso and says, "Do we touch boodoo?" We simply say, "No we don't touch boodoo" and go on about our business. It's a bit more startling in other countries, however, and can cause all sorts of cross-cultural misunderstandings. And, though most foreigners can get a drop of water on their pants and still carry on, this is intolerable to certain citizens in Schmolland who insist that the pants must come off no matter where they are, and regardless of whether another pair of pants are present.

Other families who are affected by autism are familiar and comforting to us, yet are still separate entities. Together we make up a federation of countries, kind of like Scandinavia. Like a person from Denmark talking with a person from Norway, (or in our case someone from Schmenmark talking with someone from Schmorway), we share enough similarities in our language and customs to understand each other, but conversations inevitably highlight the diversity of our traditions. "Oh your child is a runner? Mine won't go to the bathroom without asking permission." "My child eats paper. Yesterday he ate a whole video box." "My daughter only eats 4 foods, all of them white." "My son wants to blow on everyone." "My son can't stand to hear the word no. We can't use any negatives at all in our house." "We finally had to lock up the VCR because my son was obsessed with the rewind button."

There is one thing we all agree on: we are a growing population.

10 years ago, 1 in 10,000 children had autism.

Today the rate is approximately 1 in 166.

Something is dreadfully wrong. Though the causes of the increase are still being hotly debated, a number of parents and professionals believe genetic pre-disposition has collided with too many environmental insults—toxins, chemicals, anti-biotics, vaccines—to create immunological chaos in the nervous systems of developing children. One medical journalist speculated that these children are like the proverbial "canary in the coal mine" here to alert us to the growing dangers in our environment. While this is certainly not a view shared by all in the autism community, it feels true to me.

I hope that researchers discover the magic bullet we all so desperately crave. And I will never stop investigating new treatments and therapies that might help my son. But more and more my priorities are shifting from what "could be" to "what is." I look around at this country my family has created, with all its unique customs, and it feels like home. For us, any time spent "nation-building" is time well spent.

You know you are in Schmolland when...(things our children have done that we can laugh about, from the LDS_Autism group and the Autism_King (County) group in Washington)

...you're picking up the living room and you notice someone has used one of your many copies of "Procedural Safeguards for Children with Special Needs and Their Families Under IDEA (revised 7/02)" as a bookmark.

...your 6-year-old comes to you with his eyes alight, jumping up and down and screaming, "Mom, David gave me EYE CONTACT!!" (David is the non-autistic baby brother, and was only two months old at the time!)

...you don't find anything too unusual about saying, "Get your tongue up off the floor this minute!" while browsing in a scrapbook store.

...you precede sentences with the words, "Eyes on Mom" ALL the time.

...you find yourself holding your breath in the bathroom so your child won't discover you are in there and ask through the door 15 times, "Mom, are you in there?" just to hear you answer "yes" 15 times!

... you can quote state special education regulations verbatim, without any notes (chapter and verse!).

... you decide that it is better to let a child pull out an entire $1.50 spool of thread because you know the child is safely occupied for at least an hour while you finish your sewing project (LAST Easter's, that is).

... you accept ketchup as a 'vegetable.'

... you don't see any pictures on the walls because they are continually being pulled down and the glass from the frames gets broken.

... you save artwork on walls that demonstrate mastery of an ABA concept/lesson/target.

... you send rejoicing e-mails to your friends because your ASD child tried to lie to you for the first time.

... you can quote the entire script from every Disney movie ever made into video!!

....you fix dinner according to colors and textures;   buy clothes according to texture and color and you know all the words, music and lyrics to, "......................" (insert your child's favorite video).

...you are so used to giving praise to your child that you forget everyone doesn't need it. I was at the pharmacy and the old pharmacist was having such a hard time getting the sack stapled. I just stood there watching him struggle (looked familiar, sort of like my son trying to cut a straight line) and when he finally got the sack stapled, I said "Way to go, you rock!" I didn't even think before I spoke.

...you try to teach 'functions' of everything you do! We were teaching my son "functions". While I was curling my hair one morning, and he was watching me, I asked "What am I doing with this curling iron?" My son replied, "Cooking hair"....

...you sneak in to the church before the rest of your family to remove the framed prints from the walls, knowing that your son will attempt to take them down himself...again!

...you can't go to the bathroom and close the door, and your son has a fit if you flush before he can.

...you make a scrapbook page of your 10 year old tying his shoe for the first time, (having taken 4 years to do it)...

...you have to travel with a "Barney" cassette tape on a home buying trip. After days and days of driving around with the realtor and listening to Barney, you are surprised to notice that the 60 year old realtor knows how to whistle all of the Barney tunes, and he didn't even know he was doing it.

...you are in a hotel elevator and your 10 year old grabs a pop out of a man's hand, takes a sip and then dumps it, right there at his feet. YIKES!

...your autistic child pushes someone in anger and you feel like cheering because they actually realized there was someone next to them.

....your child runs up to a stranger who is walking his dog, he licks the dog, and you smile and walk away.

....everyone sees the Today Show and calls you to tell you about the new way to "cure" your child.

....your child wakes up at three in the morning laughing in the dark. You would laugh too if it weren't for the fact that it stopped being cute after two straight weeks.

...you never get to use the bathroom without being asked, "What's you doing??"

...your son brings home a permission slip from school to go to Lagoon (an amusement park called "the fun spot of Utah") and your son insists you check the NO box. Because he is afraid of the rides.

...you haunt the local thrift stores for stereos that work, knowing that your son will tear them apart the second he gets a chance.... Your neighbors give you their broken appliances so your son can tear them apart...your son owns 5 vaccums and he asks for them for his b-day and Christmas every year.....(he's 22)

..your son belches loudly then always follows up with the question, "Is that a good thing to do?"

…your daughter starts every conversation with "mom, look at me," as she's looking at everything else BUT me….

…your daughter knows when a kleenex has fallen across the room

…you commonly witness your car window rolled down and hear your daughter yell at a passing bicyclist to wear a helmet OR (better still) yells at the gruff looking man in the car next door (who also has his window rolled down) that he shouldn't smoke…

…your daughter screams at the top of her lungs in the horse barn that the people around her shouldn't talk loudly or they'll scare the horses.…

….your 5 year old daughter appears at the foot of your bed, at 4 a.m., screaming at the top of her lungs just standing with her arms out wide, so you calmly get up, push up the sleeves on her nightie so they do not touch her hands anymore and she calmly says "Thank you" and goes back to bed. (Hubby comments, "Man, this is like living with a time bomb" but is impressed with your quick response)

...you assume that EVERYONE knows who Thomas, James, Henry, Percy, Gordon, etc are.

...your son has to get up from bed to come in to let you know that "Actually, Mom, that spicy catsup from Burger King isn't so bad," SIX days after he tried it and hated it.

...when asked how the state achievement test at school is going your 4th grader with autism replies, "Fine. It puts bread on the table."

...when dining out, you order chicken fajitas which come on a sizzling, steaming plate. It is all very dramatic. When the fajitas arrive, your son sees the platter coming towards the table and leaps out of his chair yelling, "FIRE, FIRE!" , surprising everyone around. You feel very impressed with his achievement given his language and cognitive skills!

...if chanting with your hands held over your ears is a perfectly acceptable way of saying: "Thank you, I have had a lovely time but I must be going now."

And, if, on the day of his baptism, the stake primary president asks, "So, are you EXCITED today?" and your child replies (accurately) "Sister [name], you have a black 1994 Saturn SL2 twin cam with 5-speed manual transaxle!"

You might just be in Schmolland!

About the Authors:

When it comes to autism, some of the best experts are the people who live with it, either parents of kids on the spectrum, or those who are autistic. As members of the Church of Jesus Christ of Latter-day Saints, or "Mormons," we have a somewhat unique perspective which affects how we feel about autism in our lives. This book has come about through the efforts of twelve families, whose lives are touched by autism, including one chapter written by an adult who has autism himself. We have each heard time and again that this resource is badly needed, for members of the church (or of any church) and for those who work with children with autism, those who have family, friends or neighbors with autism, or anyone who wants to better understand the developmental disability. Given the current instance of autism in our society, this book may be pretty much for everyone! Our children are ranging in ages and severity of autism, so there is good information for everyone here. We have included ideas for church leaders and families as part of our own stories, since we feel that our stories provide a much-needed resource for those who are searching for ideas.

www.ingramcontent.com/pod-product-compliance
Lightning Source LLC
Chambersburg PA
CBHW030323290526
45785CB00001B/479